MW01040105

Full Name	Age & Birthday

ABOUT ME

Today I am....

☐ Happy   ☐ Bubbly   ☐ Tickled   ☐ Joyous

QUESTIONS	ANSWERS
Hair Color	
Eye Color	
Height	
Where were you born?	
Do you have any pets?	
What is your favorite food?	
Do you have any brothers and sisters?	

What do you want to be when you grow up?

What is your favorite subject in school?

What do you like to do in your free time?

What makes you unique?

Why Do Girls Get Periods?

A mother and her two young daughters sat around the kitchen table, sipping cups of tea.

The older daughter looked at her mom and said, "Mom, why do girls get periods?"

Her mom smiled and said, "That's a great question. Your period is your body's way of releasing tissue that it no longer needs. Every month, a woman's body prepares for pregnancy. Basically, girls get their periods so they can eventually become moms themselves one day. When a girl starts to get older, her body transforms in preparation for having babies."

The younger daughter piped up excitedly, "That means I have a baby in me?" Her mom laughed and shook her head.

"No, sweetheart," she said gently. "Your body isn't quite ready yet, but soon enough it will be." She explained that periods are also important because they help clear out your uterus every month, so it's healthy for when you do have children someday.

Both girls nodded with understanding and sipped their tea thoughtfully as their mom gave them reassuring smiles.

The mother continued, "These changes in hormone levels cause your body to shed the uterus lining so that a baby can grow there if you become pregnant. That's why they call it a period—it's just like a complete stop in your reproductive life cycle."

The older daughter nodded and asked, "What about cramps?" "A friend of mine gets terrible cramps sometimes."

The mom smiled and said, "That's normal too, sweetheart. Changes in hormones can cause some pain as your body adjusts to the new cycle." She went on to explain that these pains were usually manageable with over-the-counter medication and simple home remedies.

Both girls took this knowledge in with happy smiles, grateful to be more informed about their bodies and growing up.

1. Changes in _____ levels lead your body to shed the _____ of your uterus so that if you become pregnant, a baby can grow there.
   a. hormone, lining
   b. period, uterus

2. Periods are also important because every _____ they help clean out your uterus.
   a. month
   b. week

3. Period cramps are normal and manageable?
   a. True
   b. False

4. Having a period means you ARE pregnant?
   a. True
   b. False

So, What is a Period?

First, read all the way through. After that, go back and fill in the blanks. You can skip the blanks you're unsure about and finish them later. Need help? Try Google.

cramps	bleed	fertilization	Hormones	egg

Okay, so you overheard one of your pals say she got her period today, and now you're curious about it. Don't fret; we've got your back. A period is short for menstruation, the time of the menstrual cycle during which women _____. And just what is a menstrual cycle, exactly? Let's break this down!

_____ rule your menstrual cycle and direct all the bodily functions that occur during this time. The first day of your period marks the beginning of each new cycle, which may last for as long as a week. Various hormones (estradiol, luteinizing, and follicle-stimulating hormones) rise and work together to wake up the ovaries during the first two weeks.

Now things get interesting. Around day 14 of your menstrual cycle, these hormones drop, and guess what? The ovaries send an _____ down to the uterus. This is the time when the hormone progesterone starts to kick in. Its job is to thicken the lining of your uterus, just in case an egg gets fertilized by a sperm. The uterus would be all set to nourish the fertilized egg.

If no _____ occurs, progesterone falls off, and the uterus sheds its lining. This shedding causes your period, and the blood contains the remnants of the old, unused uterine lining, and the whole process starts again.

It's essential to understand your menstrual cycle patterns and be prepared for your period by having access to pads, tampons, or menstrual cups because it could start unexpectedly. Also, it's not uncommon to experience stomach _____, bloating, or mood swings during menstruation. Don't worry; there are many ways to manage the pain and discomfort that come with your period.

What's the Average Age to Start Your Period?

First, read all the way through. After that, go back and fill in the blanks. You can skip the blanks you're unsure about and finish them later. Need help? Try Google.

intimate	develops	experience	dreading	menstruation

It was a typical day in the small town of Maple Valley. The sun was shining, and birds were singing, but it was time for a very important conversation-one that mom had been _____ since her daughters started getting older.

Mom gathered her two girls, Jill and Sarah, into the living room and took a deep breath before beginning to talk about what many young women _____ at some point in their lives: starting their period.

The girls looked up with wide eyes as Mom explained what happens during _____ and why taking care of your body is essential when this natural process begins. She shared stories from when she first got her period, emphasizing how scary yet exciting it can be. Then she asked them if they had any questions about the topic or felt uncomfortable talking about it; thankfully, both girls seemed surprisingly comfortable discussing such an _____ subject!

Next, Mom wanted to ensure they knew exactly when they should expect such changes in their bodies, which vary greatly depending on age. After doing some research together online (and taking breaks for snacks!), they discovered that most girls start having periods between ages 10 and 15; however, there is no exact average age because everyone's body _____ differently over time!

Jill and Sarah left the conversation feeling confident that they now knew enough information to recognize when these changes might occur within each of them individually-significantly, if Mom or Dad could help answer any other questions along the way!

Extra Credit: What does the word menstruation means?

How Long Does a Normal Period Last

Are you wondering how long your period will last and how often it will come? Well, let me explain it to you in more detail!

First of all, your period usually lasts between two and seven days. But don't worry if it lasts a little longer or shorter than that, because everyone's body is different. Typically, the first two to three days are the heaviest, and then it gradually becomes lighter from there. So make sure to always have some pads or tampons with you, just in case!

Now, let's talk about how often you will get your period. This can be a bit tricky because your cycle might not be the same length every month. While the average cycle length is 28 days, it can actually range from 21 to 35 days. Sometimes, your period might come a little earlier or later than expected. But don't worry; this is totally normal!

In fact, your period will probably be unpredictable and irregular for the first few months. This is because your body is still adjusting to the changes happening inside of it. But after a while, you will be able to notice a pattern and figure out when your next period is coming.

One great way to track your period is by using a period-tracking app. There are lots of free ones available, which can help you track when your period is expected to arrive. This can also help you plan ahead and ensure you always have the necessary supplies.

So there you have it! Your period usually lasts between two and seven days, and might come at different times every month. But don't worry; it's all a normal part of growing up. And remember, if you ever have any questions or concerns, don't be afraid to talk to your doctor or another trusted adult.

1. Typically, your period may last anywhere from ___ to ___ days.
   a. two, seven
   b. three, six

2. The first two to three days of your menstruation are the ____.
   a. lightest
   b. heaviest

3. The typical length of a menstrual cycle is ___ days.
   a. 28
   b. 32

4. For the first few months, you may experience unpredictable and ____ bleeding.
   a. irregular
   b. regular

5. Your menstrual cycle may not occur at the same time each _____.
   a. month
   b. day

6. You'll eventually detect a ____ and figure out when your next period is due.
   a. symptoms
   b. pattern

First Period Symptoms

It was a typical Sunday afternoon in the Robinson household. Dad, Mom, and their daughter Alice were all sitting around the kitchen table discussing school and upcoming plans for the week.

Suddenly, Dad cleared his throat and looked at Alice with an expression of seriousness that caught her by surprise. He said, "Alice, your mom has already had a chat with you about periods, but I wanted to make sure you know that if there's ever anything uncomfortable or embarrassing that you want to talk about—no matter what it is —I'm here for you too."

Alice shifted uncomfortably in her chair as she tried to guess where this conversation was going. The word "period" made her feel embarrassed; she knew what they meant but still felt like she didn't have enough information on them yet.

Dad noticed her discomfort, so he softened his tone as he continued talking. "I know this can be a confusing topic, so let me explain some of the things you may experience before getting your first period. You might notice changes in mood or energy levels—feeling tired more often than usual or maybe being extra emotional—these are all normal signs."

He went on to list other symptoms such as bloating and cramps from increased hormone levels, changes in skin texture due to oil production, and spotting caused by shedding of the uterine lining during the menstrual cycle preparation stages.

By now, Alice felt much more comfortable listening in on this important lesson from Dad. She thanked him for taking time out of his day to help educate her on something that could otherwise feel awkward or embarrassing to discuss openly with parents, especially dads.

1. Before receiving your period, you might experience _____ or energy changes.
   a. mood
   b. fever

2. Who educated Alice on first-period symptoms in this story?
   a. Dad
   b. Mom

3. Period symptoms such as _____ and _____ are caused by an increase in hormone levels.
   a. blemishes, chills
   b. bloating, cramping

4. During menstrual cycle preparation, the lining of the uterus sheds, causing ____.
   a. spotting
   b. light bruising

5. Where did this story take place?
   a. at the kitchen table
   b. in Alice's bedroom

6. Early menstruation signs of increased oil production causes ____ texture changes.
   a. hair
   b. skin

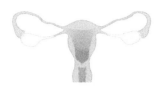

Reproductive Health Words You Should Know

Score: _____

Date: _____

Match the clues to the words. Need help? Try Google.

Across

1. A doctor who specializes in health care for the vulva, vagina, uterus, ovaries, and breasts.
2. The period of time when a fetus is developing in the womb.
4. Develops from the embryo at 10 weeks of pregnancy and receives nourishment through the placenta.
6. Chemicals that cause changes in our bodies and brains.
7. A thin, fleshy piece of tissue that stretches across part of the opening to the vagina.

Down

3. External sex and reproductive organs, like the the vulva, penis, and scrotum.
4. A benign tumor that grows on the walls of the uterus.
8. The body's natural protection against infection and disease.

IMMUNE SYSTEM
GYNECOLOGIST   HYMEN
FIBROID   HORMONES
GENITALS   FETUS
GESTATION

Breast Pain

Humans, like all mammals, have breasts. Around the start of puberty, the milk-making glands in a girl's breasts start to grow. The breasts are composed of fat and other types of tissue that encase and shield nerves, blood vessels, and milk ducts (which are little tube-like passageways).

The most important biological reason why women develop breasts is so that they can provide milk for their infants.

First, read all the way through. After that, go back and fill in the blanks. You can skip the blanks you're unsure about and finish them later.

decrease	linked	unusual	symptoms	bra

Chole was a 10th-grade girl who loved playing soccer. She had been playing on the girls' team since 8th grade and was one of the best players. However, Chole was worried about a problem that she had been having lately. She was experiencing breast pain, which was beginning to affect her game on the field. To make matters worse, her aunt passed away from breast cancer a few years ago, and she was scared it could happen to her.

Chole decided to go to her team's sports medicine doctor, Dr. McPherson. Dr. McPherson had been the team's doctor for years, and Chole had known her since the 4th grade. Dr. McPherson was a kind older lady who always had a smile on her face. Chole knew that she could trust her with her worries and concerns.

Dr. McPherson listened intently as Chole explained her _____ and concerns about breast cancer. She reassured Chole that breast pain was common for many women, especially around the time of their menstrual cycle. She explained that the pain could be caused by a _____ in hormones and suggested some tips and tricks to ease the pain. Dr. McPherson suggested that Chole cut back on salt, sugar, caffeine, and dairy, as these could be contributing factors. She also recommended that Chole wear a supportive _____ to help reduce the pain.

Dr. McPherson further explained that breast pain, although uncomfortable, is rarely linked to breast cancer. Dr. Johnson continued to explain the different types of breast pain. She learned that there are two main types: cyclic breast pain and noncyclic breast pain. Cyclic breast pain is _____ to menstrual periods; with noncyclic breast pain, the breasts themselves could be the source of the pain. Or, it could be coming from somewhere else, like nearby muscles or joints, and could be felt in the breast. She encouraged Chole to perform regular self-examinations and to see her if she noticed any _____ changes.

As Chole left Dr. McPherson, she felt relieved and hopeful. She knew that breast pain could be uncomfortable, but it wasn't something to be worried about. She was grateful to Dr. McPherson for her guidance and kindness. Chole went back to playing soccer with renewed energy and confidence. She knew she could count on Dr. McPherson for her health concerns, giving her peace of mind.

Managing a Heavy Period

For many of us, the thought of dealing with a heavy period can be overwhelming and frustrating. It's natural to worry about whether we'll leak through our tampon or pad, or if we'll even make it through the day without constant trips to the restroom. While some women experience lighter periods, others are prone to heavier cycles, known as menorrhagia.

But the question on most women's minds is: Is it normal to have heavy periods? The answer is not as simple, as everybody is different, and depending on who you ask, you might hear them say that there is no "normal" period. However, suppose you're experiencing bleeding that lasts longer than seven days, soaking through more than one pad or tampon every hour, passing blood clots larger than a quarter, or experiencing fatigue, weakness, or shortness of breath. In that case, your heavy period may be considered abnormal.

So, what qualifies as "heavy menstrual bleeding"? Generally speaking, women lose around 30–70 milliliters (mL) of menstrual blood during their periods. But when you're losing significantly more than that, it warrants concern. Losing 80 mL or more of blood per cycle or having a menstrual cycle that lasts longer than seven days are both signs of menorrhagia.

What are the symptoms of menorrhagia? Heavy menstrual bleeding is associated with numerous side effects, including fatigue, weakness, headaches, nausea, and mood changes. Women with menorrhagia may also experience stomach cramps, lower back pain, pain during intercourse, and frequent urination.

So, how can you manage heavy periods and avoid feeling overwhelmed? First, keep track of your menstrual cycle with a period tracker app, marking down when your period starts and ends and how much blood you lose each day. This will give you a clear idea of whether your bleeding exceeds the average loss of 30–70 mL per cycle. Secondly, consider using menstrual products such as period underwear, which can hold up to two tampons worth of menstrual blood, or menstrual cups, which can hold more fluid and be worn for up to 12 hours.

Aside from wearable products, medical management methods can also help. It's always best to consult your doctor to discuss these options and see which would work best for you.

Lastly, what causes heavy periods? While there is no exact cause of menorrhagia, it can be attributed to various factors such as hormonal imbalances and underlying medical conditions like thyroid dysfunction, uterine fibroids, and polyps. However, these factors may not apply to everyone, and you may be experiencing heavy periods due to other reasons like stress, poor nutrition, and lifestyle habits.

In conclusion, menorrhagia is a common issue that many women face, but there are numerous ways to manage and overcome it. By keeping track of your menstrual cycle, using wearable products, consulting with your doctor, and leading a healthy lifestyle, you can alleviate the burden of a heavy period and enjoy a more comfortable and relaxed monthly cycle. Remember that you can take care of your menstrual cycle and trust that your body can manage even the most difficult of periods without compromising your health or happiness.

1. Period blood loss averages between ___ and 70 mL for most women.
   a. 45
   b. 30

2. Heavily bleeding periods are also known as _____.
   a. menorrhagia
   b. mensuration

3. _____, poor nutrition, and unhealthy habits are all possible causes of your heavy periods.
   a. Stress
   b. Mood

4. Menorrhagia is diagnosed when a woman loses ____ mL or more of blood per cycle or has a _____-day cycle.
   a. 80, seven
   b. 30, six

Period Cramps

First, read all the way through. After that, go back and fill in the blanks. You can skip the blanks you're unsure about and finish them later. Need help? Try Google.

muscle	stretching	heating	laughing	experiencing

"Come on, sweetie," Dr. Miller said gently to the young girl sitting before him. Dr. Miller has been the young girl's doctor since she was a baby, so she knew the doctor very well. Dr. Miller said, "I know this isn't easy to talk about, but I'm here to help you."

The girl looked up at him nervously; her hands were clasped tightly together, and her eyes welled with tears. She had been _____ period cramps for some time now, but she didn't feel comfortable going to her parents or friends for help.

Dr. Miller smiled kindly at the girl before continuing his advice: "Period cramps can be tough; they're like any other kind of cramp, where a _____ contracts too hard or too fast and makes it difficult for your body to move around easily." He paused as he saw understanding slowly dawning in the girls' expression before continuing: "But there are things that you can do!" "A _____ pad is always a good idea if you have one; it helps soothe those muscles that are contracting too quickly."

He then went on to explain how exercise could also be beneficial; gentle movements such as walking or _____ would help loosen up your muscles and reduce pain levels. Then he added something that made the young girl smile: "And don't forget that even though it may not seem like it right now, _____ is actually an effective way of managing pain!" "So make sure you take some time out from all this discomforting stuff and find something funny!"

As he finished speaking, Dr. Miller's face softened into a warm smile; his words had done their job of calming down the troubled teen before him. The young girl returned his smile gratefully before hugging him goodbye and leaving with newfound confidence in tackling her period cramps head-on!

Extra Credit: List 4 things that can help ease cramps. Use Google to research your answer if needed.

_____

_____

_____

_____

CRAMPS

During your period, it is normal to have mild to significant cramps for one or two days. But many women have painful and strong menstrual cramps that can make it hard to do everyday things and exercise.

If you have very painful menstrual cramps or cramps that last longer than two or three days, make an appointment with your healthcare provider.

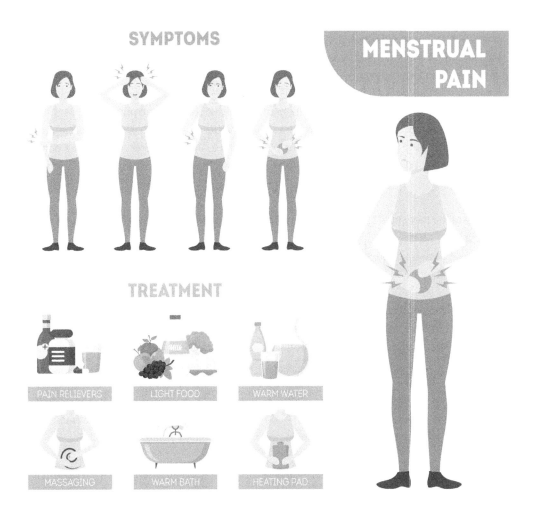

Phases of the Menstrual Cycle

First, read all the way through. After that, go back and fill in the blanks. You can skip the blanks you're unsure about and finish them later.

uterus	produce	sheds	menopause	releases

Menstruation is a normal biological process that occurs in females between puberty and _____. The menstrual cycle is divided into four phases, each with unique characteristics and functions: the follicular phase, ovulation, luteal phase, and menstruation.

Firstly, the follicular phase is the first phase of the menstrual cycle. It starts on the first day (1-14) of menstruation and lasts for approximately two weeks. During this phase, the follicles in the ovary begin to mature and _____ estrogen. The lining of the uterus also begins to thicken in preparation for a potential pregnancy. As the follicular phase progresses, one follicle becomes dominant and continues to grow, while the others shrink and die off.

The second phase of the menstrual cycle is ovulation. This phase occurs around day 14 of the menstrual cycle and lasts for about 24 to 48 hours. During ovulation, the dominant follicle _____ an egg into the fallopian tube. The egg travels through the tube towards the uterus and can be fertilized by sperm during this journey. If the egg is not fertilized, it should disintegrate within 24 hours of its release.

Following ovulation is the luteal phase, days 15-28. During this phase, the ruptured follicle transforms into the corpus luteum, which produces progesterone. Progesterone helps thicken and prepare the _____ for the potential implantation of a fertilized egg. If fertilization does not occur, the corpus luteum disintegrates, causing a drop in progesterone levels.

Lastly, menstruation is the phase that marks the end of the menstrual cycle. It typically lasts for 3-7 days, and during this phase, the thickened lining of the uterus _____, and blood and other materials exit the body through the vagina. This process is the beginning of a new menstrual cycle.

It is important to note that the length and characteristics of the menstrual cycle can vary from person to person. Certain factors like stress, illness, and weight changes can also affect the menstrual cycle.

In conclusion, the menstrual cycle is a normal biological process that occurs in females. It consists of four phases, each with unique characteristics and functions: the follicular phase, ovulation, the luteal phase, and menstruation. Understanding the menstrual cycle can help females track their menstrual cycle, monitor their health, and make informed decisions about their reproductive health.

Period Cycle Fill-in-Blanks

Score: _____

Date: _____

The lining of the uterus thickens monthly from puberty to menopause in preparation for potential pregnancy. Because of this, a fertilized egg can successfully implant in the uterus and you can get pregnant.

In a nutshell, if an egg is not implanted, the thicker tissue is shed by the body. Periods involve the monthly outflow of blood and tissue through the vagina.

The menstrual cycle is a monthly biological process that consists of several phases. Menstrual periods typically last between 21 and 40 days, while the average length is closer to 28 days.

Your cycle contains several phases that serve distinct functions and are followed by corresponding signs and symptoms.

_____

During this exercise, you will fill in the blanks with the correct word to match the definitions or clues.

hormonal	important	luteal	conception	ovulation
menstrual	bleeding	increase	follicular	cycle

1. Menstruation is an _____ part of life for teenage girls.

2. The average _____ cycle usually lasts 28 days, though this can vary from person to person.

3. During a 28-day cycle, _____ changes occur, which lead to ovulation, menstruation, and other bodily changes.

4. For teenagers, it's particularly helpful to understand menstrual _____ changes so they can better prepare themselves for what may come.

5. The first stage of the menstrual cycle is the _____ phase, where hormones are released that cause the egg in the ovary to mature.

6. The _____ phase is when a mature egg is released from the ovary into the fallopian tube and is ready for fertilization if sperm are present.

7. The third stage of the menstrual cycle is called the _____ phase.

8. During the luteal phase, hormone levels _____ to maintain a pregnancy should conception occur.

9. If no _____ occurs, then the final stage begins menstruation.

10. During menstruation, eggs, and uterine lining shed, resulting in _____ that typically lasts 3-7 days before starting over again with a new cycle beginning with the follicular phase.

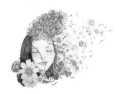

When Do Most Girls Get Their Period

In this activity, you'll see grammatical *errors*. Correct all the grammar mistakes you see.

There are **7** mistakes in this passage. 1 capital missing. 2 unnecessary capitals. 4 incorrectly spelled words.

once upon a time, a young girl named Sophie had many questions about growing up. One day she asked her mom, "Mom, when do most girls get their period?"

Her mom smiled and said, "Most girls get their period for the first tame around age 12, but it can happen earlier or later. Before your period starts, you might notice some changes In your budy, like breast growth or acne, and you might feel moody."

Sophie was happy to have her questions answered as she thought about what it would be like when her own period came. Her mom added that it could be different each month, with lighter or heavier bleeding and sometimes cramps or other PMS symptoms like headaches.

She said it's essential to take care of Sophie's body - eatang right, getting enough sleep, and exercising, and Talking to an adult she trusts about any questions she has.

"I guess I hive some things to look forward to," Sophie said with a smile.

First Visit to the Gynecologist

Monica was a shy 14-year-old girl. She had only ever been to her pediatrician and dentist, and the thought of visiting a gynecologist made her anxious. Her mom had been encouraging her to see one, especially since her menstrual cycle had started a few months ago.

She felt uneasy about the visit, not knowing what to expect. As she stepped into the gynecologist's office, she was taken aback by the sterile and unfamiliar surroundings, unlike her pediatrician's warm and friendly office.

Her heart was pounding, and her palms were sweaty as she waited for her turn to see the doctor. Her mind was swirling with questions. What would the doctor ask her? Would it hurt? Would it be embarrassing? All those thoughts made her feel vulnerable and uncomfortable.

As she sat in the consulting room, the gynecologist, Dr. Garcia, walked in. She had a warm and friendly smile that calmed Monica's nerves. Dr. Garcia asked about Monica's menstrual cycle, lifestyle and health habits, family health history, and whether she is sexually active. She answered all her questions about menstrual hygiene, sexual health, and reproductive health.

She explained, in detail, the importance of seeing a gynecologist at least once a year for early detection and prevention of any health issues. Dr. Garcia also taught Monica the importance of carrying herself with self-respect and dignity, even when confronted with obstacles in her life.

Monica was relieved that the consultation wasn't as frightening as she thought it would be. She felt a sense of empowerment and confidence that only came from taking charge of her body and health.

As Monica headed out of the clinic, she found herself walking taller and more assured than before. She knew that taking care of her body was an important part of growing up to become a healthy and responsible adult. She had learned that regular check-ups were a vital part of this and she felt optimistic and confident about her overall health.

Indeed, Monica's first visit to a gynecologist was a turning point in her life, and one that she would always look back on with gratitude. She no longer feared visiting a gynecologist, knowing that her health and well-being were more important.

Side Note: Between the ages of 13 and 15, doctors advise young women to get their first gynecological exam. Most girls have already started puberty by then, so it's an excellent time to ensure everything is growing normally.

Breast and pelvic exams are usually unnecessary for young women until they reach the age of 21. However, a pelvic exam may be performed if the doctor or nurse suspects something is wrong (or if you are experiencing symptoms such as abnormally heavy bleeding, missed periods, vaginal sores or itchiness, discharge, or other problems). Your doctor may perform a breast or pelvic examination if you have a family history of disease, especially if the disease is reproductive-related.

1. Young women under _____ rarely need breast and pelvic exams.
   a. 30
   b. 21

2. The importance of seeing a gynecologist at least _____ a year for early detection and prevention of health disorders.
   a. once
   b. twice

3. Doctors recommend a first gynecological exam for girls between _____ and ___.
   a. 16, 18
   b. 13, 15

4. Your doctor may examine your _____ or _____ if you have a family history of disease.
   a. breasts, pelvis
   b. bleeding, skin

NAME: _____

Personal Information

Full Name: _____ **SSN:** ____-____-_____
Address: _____ **DOB:** __/__/_____
City/ST/Zip: _____ **Phone:** (___) ___-_____

In Case of Emergency

Contact: _____ **Donor:** Y / N
Home #: (___) ___-_____ **Directives:** _____
Mobile #: (___) ___-_____ _____

Insurance Carrier

Company: _____ **ID #:** _____
Employer: _____ **Group #:** _____

Habits

Smoker: _____ **Drinks/WK:** _____
Blood Type: _____ **Allergies:** _____

Current Medications

Pharmacy Contact Number: (___) ___-_____

Name	Description	Dosage	Purpose

Vitamins/Food Supplements

Name	Description	Dosage	Purpose

Known Conditions, Events, and Previous Surgeries

Date	Event

Current Physicians

Type	Name	Number

Annual physical exam requirements may vary depending on where you live and school. This form gives you an idea of what info a doctor might share with the school about a student.

PRIVATE PHYSICIAN'S REPORT OF PHYSICAL EXAMINATION OF A PUPIL OF SCHOOL AGE

DATE _____ 20_____

NAME OF SCHOOL _____ GRADE _____ HOMEROOM _____

NAME OF CHILD			DATE OF BIRTH	SEX
				☐ ☐
Last	First	Middle		M F

ADDRESS

_____

| No. and Street | City or Post Office | Borough or Township | County | State | Zip Code |

MEDICAL HISTORY IMMUNIZATIONS AND TESTS

VACCINE	Enter Month, Day, and Year each immunization was given DOSES			BOOSTERS & DATES	
Diphtheria and Tetanus (Circle): DTaP, DTP, DT, TD	1 / /	2 / /	3 / /	4 / /	5 / /
Polio (Circle): OPV, IPV	1 / /	2 / /	3 / /	4 / /	5 / /
Measles, Mumps, Rubella	1 / /	2 / /			
Hepatitis B	1 / /	2 / /	3 / /		
HIB	1 / /	2 / /	3 / /		
Varicella	1 / /	2 / /	Varicella Disease or Lab Evidence Date: _____		
Other: _____					

☐ MEDICAL EXEMPTION   The physical condition of the above named child is such that immunization would endanger life or health
☐ RELIGIOUS EXEMPTION (Includes a strong moral or ethical conviction similar to a religious belief and requires a written
     statement from the parent/guardian)

If Applicable:

Tuberculin Tests Date Applied	Arm	Device	Antigen	Manufacturer	Signature
Date Read	Results (mm)		Signature		

Follow-Up of significant tuberculin tests:
Parent/Guardian notified of significant findings on _____.

Result of Diagnostic Studies: _____.
Preventive Anti-Tuberculosis – Chemotherapy ordered. ☐   ☐   _____
                                                      No   Yes   Date

Dental Health History Form Practice

Dental history reviews the patient's past dental experiences and current dental issues. A look at the dental history can often tell you about past dental problems, previous dental treatment, and how the patient has responded to treatment.

Patient Name: _____   Date: _____

Email Address: _____   Phone No. _____

Address: _____

Medications: _____
_____

Allergies: _____
_____

Pregnant: ☐ Yes ☐ No   Nursing: ☐ Yes ☐ No

Alcohol Use: ☐ Never ☐ Occasionally ☐ Monthly ☐ Weekly ☐ Daily ☐ 4+ per Day

Smoking: ☐ Never ☐ Occasionally ☐ 1 per Day ☐ 1 Pack per Day ☐ 2+ Packs per Day

Illegal Drug Use: ☐ Never ☐ Occasionally ☐ Monthly ☐ Weekly ☐ Daily

Exercise: ☐ Never ☐ Occasionally ☐ Weekly ☐ 2-3 Times per Week ☐ Daily

Dental Symptoms		
Pain in teeth	☐ Yes	☐ No
Teeth sensitivity	☐ Yes	☐ No
Teeth sensitivity to heat	☐ Yes	☐ No
Teeth sensitivity to cold	☐ Yes	☐ No
Teeth sensitivity to sour	☐ Yes	☐ No
Teeth sensitivity to sweet	☐ Yes	☐ No
Bleeding gums	☐ Yes	☐ No
Bleeding gums after flossing	☐ Yes	☐ No
Sensitive gums	☐ Yes	☐ No
Swollen gums	☐ Yes	☐ No
Headaches	☐ Yes	☐ No
Earaches	☐ Yes	☐ No
Jaw aching	☐ Yes	☐ No
Tired jaw	☐ Yes	☐ No
Clicking jaw	☐ Yes	☐ No
Jaw gets stuck	☐ Yes	☐ No
Unable to totally open mouth	☐ Yes	☐ No
TMJ	☐ Yes	☐ No
Clenched jaw	☐ Yes	☐ No
Grinding teeth	☐ Yes	☐ No
Food catches in teeth	☐ Yes	☐ No
Tongue pain	☐ Yes	☐ No
Tongue swelling	☐ Yes	☐ No
	☐ Yes	☐ No
	☐ Yes	☐ No
	☐ Yes	☐ No
	☐ Yes	☐ No

Dental History		
I gag easily	☐ Yes	☐ No
Dental work makes me nervous	☐ Yes	☐ No
I brush _____ times per day		
I floss _____ times per day		
I use mouthwash _____ times per day		
I chew gum regularly	☐ Yes	☐ No
I chew tobacco regularly	☐ Yes	☐ No
I smoke a pipe regularly	☐ Yes	☐ No
I take pain relievers often	☐ Yes	☐ No
I take muscle relaxants often	☐ Yes	☐ No
I take antidepressants often	☐ Yes	☐ No
I have had trauma to the head	☐ Yes	☐ No
I have had trauma to the face	☐ Yes	☐ No
I have had trauma to the ear	☐ Yes	☐ No
I have had trauma to the mouth	☐ Yes	☐ No
I have had trauma to the throat	☐ Yes	☐ No
I take fluoride supplements	☐ Yes	☐ No
I am dissatisfied with my teeth	☐ Yes	☐ No
I wear dentures	☐ Yes	☐ No
I have braces	☐ Yes	☐ No
I don't like the color of my teeth	☐ Yes	☐ No
I want total dental care	☐ Yes	☐ No
	☐ Yes	☐ No
	☐ Yes	☐ No
	☐ Yes	☐ No
	☐ Yes	☐ No

The medical record information release (HIPAA) form lets a patient allow any person or 3rd party to have access to their health records.

AUTHORIZATION FOR RELEASE OF HEALTH INFORMATION

Patient Name _____ **Date of Birth** _____

The above named person must indicate when this authorization is to expire:
☐ When information is received   ☐ In one year
☐ In six months   ☐ In three years
☐ On date _____

The person named above is or has been a patient of
Name of Person,
Provider, or Facility _____
Address _____
Phone _____
Fax _____

The person named above hereby authorizes _____ **to**
Name of Person, Provider, or Facility

☐ Request health information from   ☐ Send health information to
☐ Discuss health information with   ☐ Discuss health information with

The person named above authorizes information to be requested or released by representatives of
Name Of Person,
Provider, Or Facility _____
Address _____
_____
Phone _____
Fax _____

Scope
☐ All information regarding assessment, diagnosis, and treatment of patient's condition, concern, or disease (specify):
_____

☐ All information regarding care received
by patient between the dates of _____ and _____
                                                            Starting Date   Ending Date
☐ Other information (specify):

Authorization

_____
Printed name of Patient or Authorized Representative

_____   _____   _____   _____
Signature of Patient   Date   Signature of witness   Date
or Authorized Representative

If not signed by the patient, indicate relationship of authorizing person to patient:

☐ Parent or guardian of minor child
☐ Guardian or conservator of conserved patient
☐ Beneficiary or personal Representative of a deceased individual

Certain information is protected further and requires special authorization. The individual named above must initial and date each item to allow its dissemination or discussion. Without initialing and dating an item, the information contained within, if any, cannot be disseminated or discussed.

Initial	Date		From	To
_____	_____	Alcohol or Drug Use/Abuse Treatment	_____	_____
_____	_____	Mental Health Treatment	_____	_____
_____	_____	HIV Status or Treatment	_____	_____

The above named person has the following rights:

• This authorization is valid just for the health care information requested and authorized above. You may obtain a copy of this authorization form by contacting us.

• This authorization will be valid till the date specified above. Additionally, you may cancel this authorization at any moment by contacting this clinic or caretaker in writing. Your revocation shall be recognized except to the extent that you behaved in good faith while the agreement was in effect.

• You have the right to inspect the information whose re-release you are allowing. This and other specific rights concerning the management of your health information are detailed in our document on Privacy Practices.

• The recipient of the information you are authorizing may re-release or disclose it. Such extra disclosures or releases may be permissible under applicable legislation. We are not liable for the activities of third parties who may get information as a result of this authorization.

• You have the option of refusing to sign this authorization. This denial will have no effect on your ability to seek treatment, save to the extent that the information asked will aid your health care practitioner in identifying the most suitable course of action. Your failure to sign this authorization will have no effect on your benefit eligibility.

PLEASE NOTE: Unless otherwise required by law, we will only distribute material prepared by our employees or agents, such as chart notes, lab findings, summaries, and consultation reports. The records of other providers, hospitals, and other care facilities must be requested directly from those providers or facilities themselves.

There may be a charge for copying your records. If the information is for personal use, you are entitled to one complimentary copy of your personal health information record. Additional copies for you, future distributions to you, and distributions to other providers, persons, or facilities may be subject to a reasonable fee. For additional information on applicable copying fees, please contact the clinic's office manager or site administrator.

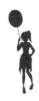

Can I Skip My Period?

First, read all the way through. After that, go back and fill in the blanks. You can skip the blanks you're unsure about and finish them later. Need help? Try Google.

menopause	summer	remedies	nature	methods

Kim was so excited about her upcoming sweet sixteen pool party. She had been planning it all _____, from the decorations to the perfect playlist. But now that the day was almost here, she had a problem-she didn't want to start her period on her birthday!

She decided to take matters into her own hands and asked around for advice on how to skip it. Her friends told her about a few different _____ they had heard about on social media, but Kim wasn't sure if they were safe or reliable, so she chose not to try them out.

She called up her grandmother, a wise woman in her seventies who was known for having natural _____ for any ailment. Unfortunately, Kim didn't get the response she hoped for. Granny told Kim that certain forms of hormonal birth control could enable a woman to skip her period. However, besides that, it wasn't safe or proven to stop your period outside of pregnancy or _____. Granny wasn't too keen on this idea and again advised against it: "Kim, it is not safe or healthy for you at your age," Granny said firmly but kindly. "Let nature take its course." Granny then warned Kim against taking medical advice from social media and her friends as well.

Kim reluctantly accepted this advice but still felt disappointed that she wouldn't have a "perfect" birthday without being on her period. As days passed leading up to the party, though, something strange happened-miraculously enough, by some divine intervention perhaps, when it came time for Kim's birthday party: there was no sign of Aunt Flo! It seemed like _____ had taken its own course after all-just as Granny said it would!

The rest of the night went off without a hitch, and everyone enjoyed themselves tremendously! When Kim thanked Granny later that week over a Skype call (since Granny didn't make it to her party), Granny just winked with a smile and said, "Grandmother knows best!"

Extra Credit: (1.) What did Kim's Granny advise her about skipping her period? (2.) What does the word menopause mean? Use Google to research your answer if needed.

....

....

....

Reproductive Health Words You Should Know

Score: _____

Date: _____

Match the clues to the words. Need help? Try Google.

Across

3. The process of childbirth.
5. The first time a person gets their period.
7. A breast/chest cancer screening that takes x-rays of the breasts/chest tissue to find lumps.
8. The tightening and releasing of the muscles that stop urination in order to prevent and improve urinary incontinence.
9. The inability to become pregnant or to cause a pregnancy.

Down

2. A treatment that prevents cervical cancer.
4. The lips of the vulva.
5. A health care provider who is trained to assist in childbirth.
6. Menstrual bleeding that's heavier or longer lasting than usual.
9. Being unable to control urination or bowel movements.

LABOR   LABIA   INFERTILITY
MAMMOGRAM
MENORRHAGIA   MIDWIFE
INCONTINENCE   LEEP
MENARCHE   KEGEL
EXERCISES

Dark Red Period Blood

In this activity, you'll see grammatical *errors*. Correct all the grammar mistakes you see.

There are **9** mistakes in this passage. 1 capital missing. 2 unnecessary capitals. 6 incorrectly spelled words.

Carla was fealing a bit anxious. She had just started her period, and the blood on her pad wasn't red like she expected. Instead, it was black. she was a nervous wreck-after all, something must have gone wrong if the color of her menstrual bloud looked so strange!

She decided to ask someone who would know more than her: Aunt Kelly, who is a nurse by profession. Carla nervously explained what happened and asked why this could be happening to her body.

Aunt Kelly calmly replied that it's normal for period blood to sometimes Be dark brown or even black at the beginning or end of your cycle. When flow is slow during these tames, old blood can get exposed to oxygen, which causes iron in the blood cells to oxidize and become darker. But she added that if menstrual bleeding stays black throughout an Entire cycle, there may be cause for concern! She told Carla not to hesitate to tell her mom and contact a healthcare provider should anything else seam off with regard to menstruation health from that point forward; better safe than sorry!

Carla felt relieved after hearing Aunt Kelly's explanation but also empowered knowing she now had all the necessary informatoin about what happens when you start your period, including having insight into why one might experience different colors of menstrual floid occasionally over time!

Reproductive Health Words You Should Know

Match the clues to the words. Need help? Try Google.

Across

2. Medicines that are used to cure infections caused by bacteria.
4. Not having sex.
5. The narrow, lower part of the uterus, with a small opening connecting the uterus to the vagina.
6. The reproductive cell stored in the ovaries and released during ovulation.
7. The organism that develops from a pre-embryo during the second month of pregnancy.

Down

1. The period of physical and emotional change between the beginning of puberty and early adulthood.
2. The dark area surrounding the nipple.
8. The ability to have children or cause a pregnancy.

EMBRYO   AREOLA
ADOLESCENCE   CERVIX
FERTILITY   ANTIBIOTICS
EGG   CELIBACY

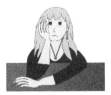

What happens during PMS?

Today, we will talk about something that affects almost every woman at some point in her life: PMS or Premenstrual Syndrome. PMS is a complex group of symptoms that affect women during the luteal phase of their menstrual cycle, which is the period between ovulation and menstruation.

PMS is a collection of physical and emotional symptoms that occur in the week leading up to your period. Hormonal fluctuations in your body cause it as your ovaries prepare to release an egg. These hormonal changes can affect the levels of serotonin, a chemical in the brain that regulates mood, appetite, and sleep.

So, what are the most common symptoms of PMS? Well, there are a few, and they can range from mild bloating and mood swings to severe cramping and headaches. Some of the most common PMS symptoms include:

1. Mood swings
2. Breast tenderness
3. Bloating
4. Acne breakouts
5. Fatigue
6. Headaches
7. Cravings
8. Insomnia
9. Irritability and anxiety

If you're experiencing any of these symptoms, don't worry; you can do several things to help ease them. Here are some tips:

1. Exercise regularly
2. Reduce your salt and sugar intake
3. Eat a balanced diet rich in vitamins, minerals, and healthy fats and drink plenty of water
4. Take painkillers, such as ibuprofen or acetaminophen, for pain relief
5. Use heat therapy for abdominal cramps, such as a hot water bottle or warm towel
6. Practice relaxation techniques, such as yoga, meditation, or deep breathing

But why do we experience PMS, you may ask? Well, the exact cause of PMS isn't known yet, but medical researchers think it has something to do with the changes in hormones during the menstrual cycle. Hormones such as estrogen and progesterone help regulate our menstrual cycle and influence our mood, energy levels, and physical health. When there's an imbalance of these hormones during the luteal phase, it can lead to the various symptoms of PMS.

To summarize, PMS is a group of symptoms that can affect women during the luteal phase of their menstrual cycle. Symptoms can range from mild to severe. While the exact cause isn't known, you can do things to ease PMS symptoms, such as exercise and eating a balanced diet. Remember, it's all part of being a woman, and with these tips, you'll be able to manage your PMS symptoms without letting them interfere with your daily life.

1. PMS is characterized by a number of _____ and _____ symptoms.

    a. monthly cycles, bleeding

    b. physical, emotional

2. What does the acronym PMS mean?

    a. Premenstrual Syndrome

    b. Premedical Symptoms

3. Serotonin is a _____ in the brain that affects mood, hunger, and sleep.

    a. chemical

    b. tissue

4. _____ and progesterone are two hormones that help control our monthly cycle.

    a. Melatonin

    b. Estrogen

PMDD

Typically, you're a fairly laid-back person. Things don't typically affect you much. However, today you wake up feeling sluggish and bloated. You are one week away from your period. You were unable to slumber last night. You are late for school due to oversleeping, and none of your jeans fit. Because your mother is telling you to hurry up, you scream at her. The door of your locker is stuck and you have a pimple. It appears to be much more difficult to focus in class. You sob uncontrollably when someone tells you that you appear exhausted. You cry because of cramps in gym class, and you yell at your closest friend for no apparent reason. The universe stinks and nothing goes right. Normally, you would want to hang out with your friends to feel better, but today you just want to curl up on the sofa and devour a pint of Ben and Jerry's.

It's possible that you have premenstrual dysphoric disorder if this happens to you every month around the same time. PMDD, which stands for premenstrual dysphoric disorder, is a more serious form of PMS. People with PMDD experience intense mood and physical changes each month before their period, which lessen once their period begins. With PMS, mood fluctuations, cramps, and food cravings may only last a few days, but with PMDD, they may last up to two weeks.

If you have PMDD, you feel normal throughout the entire month until approximately 7 to 10 days before your period begins.

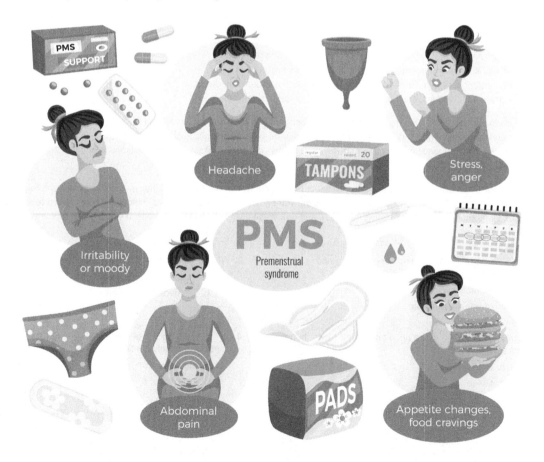

2 Periods in One Month

A menstrual cycle is defined as the time between the start of one menstrual period and the start of the next.

Your menstrual cycles may be irregular and hard to predict for the first few years after you've had your first period.

It's true that every woman's menstruation is different. While some women may bleed for up to a week, others may only bleed for two. Your period could be very light and scarcely noticed, or it could be quite heavy and cause you discomfort. You may or may not get cramps, and if you do, they may be mild to severe.

If your periods have been quite regular, you generally don't have anything to worry about. However, you should be on the lookout for any oddities in your monthly menstrual cycle.

_____

First, read all the way through. After that, go back and fill in the blanks. You can skip the blanks you're unsure about and finish them later.

hormones	cycles	irregular	uterine	periods

Tina was a junior in high school and had been experiencing something strange with her _____. She would have them twice in the same month, which seemed to be happening more often. She knew that wasn't normal, so one day, she decided to go talk to the nurse at her school about it.

When she arrived, she felt relieved that someone else might finally understand what was going on. As soon as they started talking, the nurse explained how having menstrual _____ 21 days apart could lead to having two periods per month; however, this could also indicate other health issues, such as ovarian cysts, endometriosis, _____ fibroids, pelvic inflammatory disease, and cervical neoplasia. Tina thought back over the past few months, trying to remember if there had been any other signs of anything being wrong, but nothing had come up for her until now.

The nurse told Tina not to worry too much yet but told her to see a doctor in case something important was going on under all those _____ and bleeding cycles. With a smile of understanding, Tina thanked the nurse for her time and felt much better about her situation.

Tina made an appointment with her doctor right away because, although _____ bleeding can sometimes be normal during puberty, it's essential not to take any risks when it comes to your body's health!

Why Is My Period Late?

Your period should begin between 21 and 35 days after your last period if you don't have a medical issue that affects your menstrual cycle. Regular periods can vary. If your normal menstrual cycle is 28 days and you haven't had your period by day 29, your period is considered late.

First, read all the way through. After that, go back and fill in the blanks. You can skip the blanks you're unsure about and finish them later.

pregnancy	diet	research	overnight	anxious

Samantha had been feeling off for weeks. She was tired, her stomach hurt constantly, and she felt _____ all the time. But now that it was almost June, another thing had started to bother her: why was her period late? As Samantha tried to figure out what could be causing this, she decided it was best to talk to someone about it.

She knew one person who would know how to handle the situation: her cool older sister, Lily. Lily always seemed so wise beyond her years, and Samantha trusted her opinion more than anyone else's. So when they were alone in their room that night, Samantha nervously asked, "Why is my period late?"

Lily immediately smiled reassuringly and pulled out a notebook from underneath her bed. Inside were pages upon pages of notes from medical journals she read as part of _____ projects for school (she wanted to be a doctor someday). After explaining some possible causes like stress, _____ change, or being under the weather-which made sense given how things had been going lately-she then mentioned _____ as an unlikely but still potential cause.

Samantha thanked Lily for the new information before getting ready for bed with new knowledge in hand and hope in her heart; everything would ultimately work itself out just fine! Samantha now realizes that these problems won't go away _____, and that's okay, too!

Extra Credit: What are irregular periods? Use Google to research.

_____

_____

_____

_____

Vaginal Discharge

Vaginal discharge, as uncomfortable and embarrassing as it may seem, is an entirely normal and healthy process that happens to all girls and women with vaginas. It's a fluid that comes from the vagina and helps clean and moisturize it while also protecting against infections.

Some of you may have noticed this on the toilet paper when you wipe or in your underwear. That's because it's perfectly normal for the quantity, texture, and color of the discharge to change throughout the month, depending on your menstrual cycle. However, some changes in discharge can signal a problem, indicating that it's time to consult your doctor.

Normal vaginal discharge can vary in color, texture, and amount between different individuals, depending on several factors such as age, menstrual cycle, pregnancy, or even stress levels. However, it's essential to identify what's usual for your body to notice when something is out of the ordinary and seek medical advice if necessary.

Generally speaking, normal vaginal discharge should be clear, white, or off-white in color, and it shouldn't smell unpleasant, burn, itch, or cause irritation. It's also common for some girls to have a more substantial amount of vaginal discharge than others, which might require wearing a pantyliner to keep their underwear dry. On the other hand, some girls do not have much discharge at all, which can also be entirely normal.

When it comes to the texture of the discharge, it can vary from thin, sticky, and elastic to a thick, gooey consistency, depending on the menstrual cycle phase. For instance, the discharge can become more stretchy and slippery during ovulation, allowing the sperm to swim more easily. Toward the end of the menstrual cycle, the discharge can become slightly thicker and stickier to form a plug that prevents infection from entering the cervix.

However, some changes in the discharge may indicate a problem that requires medical attention. For instance, if the discharge is yellow or green, has a strong smell, appears curdled or cottage cheese-like, or comes with itching, burning, or pain, it might indicate an infection. Yeast (candidiasis), bacteria (bacterial vaginosis), or sexually transmitted infections (STIs) like chlamydia or gonorrhea are some of the most common causes of vaginal infections.

In conclusion, vaginal discharge is a natural and normal process that varies from person to person and throughout the menstrual cycle. It's essential to know what's typical for your body to identify any changes that might signal an infection, especially if they are accompanied by discomfort or odor. If you suspect an infection, don't hesitate to speak to your parent(s) or a healthcare provider, who can diagnose and treat the problem if necessary. Remember, taking care of your vaginal health is essential to maintaining overall well-being, and it starts with awareness and education.

1. Vaginal discharge should be clear, white, or off-white, and _____.
   a. odorless
   b. slight smell

2. Depending on the menstrual cycle phase, the discharge might be thin, sticky, elastic, or _____ and gooey.
   a. thick
   b. bloody

3. At the end of the menstrual cycle, the discharge might thicken and cling to the _____, preventing infection.
   a. cervix
   b. vagina

4. Some girls need a _____ to keep their underwear dry because they have more vaginal discharge than others.
   a. tampon
   b. pantyliner

5. If the discharge is yellow or green, smells unpleasant, looks curdled or cottage cheese-like, itches, burns, or hurts, it may be an _____.
   a. infection
   b. pregnancy

6. Vaginal infections are often caused by _____, bacteria, or STIs like chlamydia or gonorrhea.
   a. birth control
   b. yeast

Yeast Infection

First, read all the way through. After that, go back and fill in the blanks. You can skip the blanks you're unsure about and finish them later.

unscented	urine	inflammation	medical	itching

Trina was working the Friday evening shift at the local movie theatre. She had been feeling discomfort and _____ around her vagina for a few days but hadn't thought much about it until that night. On her break, Trina went to the bathroom and noticed that she was red, and there appeared to be some irritation on her skin. She immediately called her best friend Lisa in a panic, asking, "How can I tell if I have a yeast infection?"

Lisa cracked an inappropriate joke instead of answering: "Why did the rich woman sell yeast? Then Lisa giggled and said, "To raise some dough." Trina wasn't amused by this joke (not even finding it remotely funny). Lisa then told Trina that she wasn't sure because she never had one before and that she should seek _____ advice as soon as possible so they could diagnose her correctly.

Trina couldn't get an appointment with her primary physician until Monday, so instead, she went to the weekend clinic where her mom worked for help on Saturday morning. When she arrived, Trina told them what had been going on. After noting down all of her symptoms and collecting a _____ sample, the doctor informed Trina that although the itching suggested it could be a yeast infection, luckily for her, it wasn't one! Instead, he concluded that it was likely due to an allergic reaction from recently using new soap or detergent, which had caused the irritation. Tina then remembered that she was using this new body wash she received last month as a Christmas gift.

The doctor also educated Trina further; he advised that yeast infections can cause a vaginal discharge that resembles cottage cheese and is thick and white. The discharge can be watery and often smell-less. He continued and said that, usually, to check for _____ and discharge; most doctors will perform a pelvic exam. With a cotton swab, a doctor can collect a sample of the discharge coming from the patient's vagina. From there, the sample will be examined under a microscope to determine whether the patient has a yeast infection. He added that the pelvic exam wasn't necessary in her case because she had no other symptoms. And in the future, he said, use a mild, _____ soap or plain water. Using a new body wash, especially one with fragrance, can disturb the pH of your vagina and cause irritation or a yeast infection.

Trina thanked the doctor for his help and left after hearing this news. She has learned her lesson and will take extra precautions to maintain her personal hygiene in the future to avoid similar incidents.

Different Menstrual Products

First, read all the way through. After that, go back and fill in the blanks. You can skip the blanks you're unsure about and finish them later.

string	absorbent	base	inserted	rayon

When young women have their first period, it is essential that they know there are different menstrual products available to them. Let's explore the variety of menstrual products that can cater to their different preferences and needs.

Sanitary Pads

Sanitary pads, or napkins, are the most commonly used menstrual product. They are attached to the inside of the woman's underwear and work by absorbing menstrual blood through layers of absorbent material like _____, cotton, and plastic. Over the decades, the design of pads has evolved to become much more absorbent and comfortable, with a wide range available to suit different flows.

Tampons

Tampons are a popular option, which absorbs menstrual blood internally through vaginal insertion. Tampons can take practice, and not everyone finds them comfortable to use. They can be left in for about four hours, at which point they are removed by pulling gently on the _____. Leaks are common with tampons, so an additional pantiliner may be required.

Menstrual Cups

In recent years, many people have given up the more traditional options of tampons and pads in favor of the menstrual cup. This small silicone or latex cup works by being folded and _____ internally, where it collects blood. They are a sustainable option since they can last for years with proper care. Menstrual cups take some time to get positioning right, but once the technique is mastered, leakages shouldn't be a problem, and they are comfortable and safe to use.

Menstrual Discs

The lesser-known menstrual disc, made of plastic or silicone, is also inserted into the vagina and rests on the _____ of the cervix. It can stay in for up to 12 hours and works by collecting blood in the disc. Menstrual discs can take some time to figure out how to use correctly, but they offer a sustainable and comfortable option.

Period Underwear

The latest newcomer to the period scene is period underwear. They look like regular underwear but have a special _____ layer that prevents clothing leakage. As they are washable and reusable, they are one of the most sustainable options available. A good pair of period underwear will prevent odors, making them comfortable and discreet to the wearer.

It's essential for young women to experiment with different menstrual products and find the ones that are right for them. Each product has pros and cons, so choosing the one that suits their lifestyle and preferences is important. Changing them regularly and maintaining good hygiene to avoid infections is essential no matter what product they use. By knowing about the different menstrual products available, young women can take control of their menstrual cycle and lead a healthy, active life.

Choosing Products

It can be overwhelming to shop for period products.

Whether you're getting ready for your first period or just want to try something new, the market today is full of choices for all body types, sizes, lifestyles, flows, budgets, and environmental preferences.

Explaining the basics

1. **Tampons** are one of the most common items for women who have their periods, but not everyone can use them.

2. If you don't like tampons, you can use **pads i**nstead.

3. If you want to save money and help the environment by making less trash, look for reusable choices like menstrual cups, discs, and **period underwear.**

4. If you don't want to use period underwear or reusable pads, **menstrual cups** are a newer choice that is becoming more and more popular.

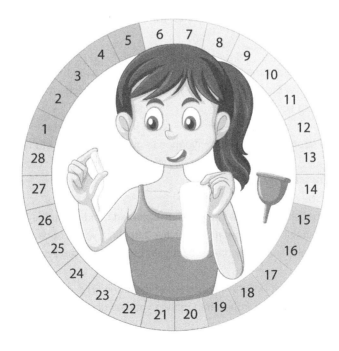

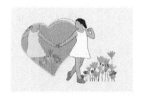

Body Image and Self-Esteem

First, read all the way through. After that, go back and fill in the blanks. You can skip the blanks you're unsure about and finish them later.

unique	yoga	reel	influencers	societal
catty	mood	experimenting	complimented	boost
confident	healthier	negativity	dark	incorporating
low	thoughts	affirmations	sleep	beauty

Tiffany struggled with body image and self-esteem issues throughout her teenage years. She felt as though every glance in the mirror brought with it a wave of self-doubt and criticism. She compared herself to the models and _____ she saw on social media, feeling that she would never measure up.

The teasing and _____ remarks from her peers did not help. It took a lot of work to keep up with the superficial trends of her generation. Tiffany felt as though she was drowning in expectations and insecurities.

One day, Tiffany's counselor, Mrs. Bradley, noticed she looked crestfallen as she walked by the counselor's office. Mrs. Bradley called her in for a chat, and soon Tiffany was pouring out her struggles with her body image and _____ self-worth. Mrs. Bradley listened with compassion, understanding the immense pressures teenagers face these days.

She told Tiffany that she wasn't alone in her struggles. Every individual goes through phases where they are uncomfortable with their body. Mrs. Bradley then gave Tiffany practical advice on accepting herself for who she is rather than trying to keep up with societal _____ standards.

Tiffany began to adopt these strategies, and her confidence began to grow. She started to buy clothes that suited her body type while _____ with different hairstyles and accessories. Slowly but surely, she began to see her reflection in the mirror with new eyes.

Feeling more comfortable in her skin, Tiffany's self-esteem improved rapidly. Her friends and even strangers _____ her, and she started to get more positive attention, which boosted her morale. Soon enough, she got asked to the school's Valentine's Day dance by a cute boy she had always admired from afar.

With newfound confidence, Tiffany felt like she was on top of the world. The moral of the story is to be body positive and love yourself for who you are rather than putting yourself under immense pressure to fit in with _____ beauty standards.

Tiffany learned to appreciate her _____ attributes and embrace her identity. She felt empowered to be herself and began living life on her terms. The world can be a _____ place, but with a positive mindset and self-love, anything is possible.

Tips to Improve Body Image and Self-Esteem

Body image and self-esteem are closely interrelated and can impact how individuals feel about themselves. Although a negative body image is a common struggle for many people, it can be improved by _____ some of these practical and actionable tips.

Practice Self-Care: Pamper yourself with small acts of self-care each day, such as taking a relaxing bath, getting enough _____, and doing things you enjoy. They don't have to be expensive or elaborate, but focus on activities that bring joy and comfort.

Start Your Day Positively: Begin your day positively by saying _____ and stating your intentions. For example, "I am confident in my own skin and love myself just the way I am" can set the tone for your day in a positive way.

Surround Yourself with Positivity: Spend time with people who make you feel good about yourself and avoid people that bring _____ or criticism into your life.

Stay Active: Physical activity, such as cycling, running, or _____, boosts mood and confidence as it interacts with endorphins. Even a small amount of physical exercise can help you feel energized, happy and help to eliminate body negativity.

Find Your Own Style: Dress up in clothing and colors that make you feel comfortable and _____. Dressing up for yourself, not necessarily for others, can help you be more comfortable and feel beautiful in your skin.

Positive Self-Talk: Practice positive self-talk by replacing negative _____ with positive affirmations, as mentioned above. Instead of having negative self-talk, say, "I am beautiful and capable of anything" to yourself throughout the day.

Avoid Comparing Yourself to Others: Accept your own unique attributes, and avoid comparing yourself to others on social media. Remember that social media is just curated content; what people show online is their highlight _____, not necessarily the reality.

Eat Healthily: Healthy eating can directly impact our health, _____, and self-esteem. Understanding what your body needs and making better dietary choices is essential.

Celebrate Your Accomplishments: Celebrate your successes, no matter how small, by rewarding yourself or acknowledging them. It will encourage positive self-talk, _____ your self-esteem, and improve your overall mood.

It's essential to remember that change takes time and requires patience. By incorporating these tips, you can build _____ habits and create a positive outlook for your body and self-esteem.

SKIN CARE

A skin response called progestogen hypersensitivity usually happens when a woman is having her period. Symptoms generally start 3–10 days before a woman's period and go away when her period is over. Some of the things that can happen to the skin are rashes, bumps, itching, hives, and red, flaky spots.

Changes in hormones can cause skin problems like acne and localized spots or itching of the skin (called neurodermatitis). But more often than not, underlying skin problems like eczema, psoriasis, or cold spots can get worse right before a woman's period.

SKINCARE ROUTINE CONCEPTS

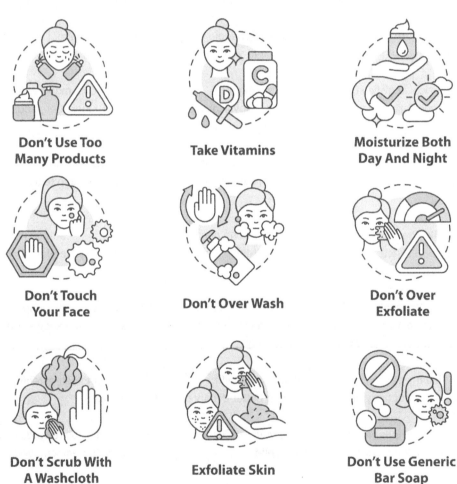

Don't Use Too Many Products

Take Vitamins

Moisturize Both Day And Night

Don't Touch Your Face

Don't Over Wash

Don't Over Exfoliate

Don't Scrub With A Washcloth

Exfoliate Skin

Don't Use Generic Bar Soap

Why Do Girls Get Periods?

A mother and her two young daughters sat around the kitchen table, sipping cups of tea.

The older daughter looked at her mom and said, "Mom, why do girls get periods?"

Her mom smiled and said, "That's a great question. Your period is your body's way of releasing tissue that it no longer needs. Every month, a woman's body prepares for pregnancy. Basically, girls get their periods so they can eventually become moms themselves one day. When a girl starts to get older, her body transforms in preparation for having babies."

The younger daughter piped up excitedly, "That means I have a baby in me?" Her mom laughed and shook her head.

"No, sweetheart," she said gently. "Your body isn't quite ready yet, but soon enough it will be." She explained that periods are also important because they help clear out your uterus every month, so it's healthy for when you do have children someday.

Both girls nodded with understanding and sipped their tea thoughtfully as their mom gave them reassuring smiles.

The mother continued, "These changes in hormone levels cause your body to shed the uterus lining so that a baby can grow there if you become pregnant. That's why they call it a period—it's just like a complete stop in your reproductive life cycle."

The older daughter nodded and asked, "What about cramps?" "A friend of mine gets terrible cramps sometimes."

The mom smiled and said, "That's normal too, sweetheart. Changes in hormones can cause some pain as your body adjusts to the new cycle." She went on to explain that these pains were usually manageable with over-the-counter medication and simple home remedies.

Both girls took this knowledge in with happy smiles, grateful to be more informed about their bodies and growing up.

---

1. Changes in ____ levels lead your body to shed the ____ of your uterus so that if you become pregnant, a baby can grow there.
- a. hormone, lining
- b. period, uterus

2. Periods are also important because every ____ they help clean out your uterus.
- a. month
- b. week

3. Period cramps are normal and manageable?
- a. True
- b. False

4. Having a period means you ARE pregnant?
- a. True
- b. False

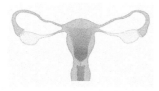

So, What is a Period?

First, read all the way through. After that, go back and fill in the blanks. You can skip the blanks you're unsure about and finish them later. Need help? Try Google.

cramps	bleed	fertilization	Hormones	egg

Okay, so you overheard one of your pals say she got her period today, and now you're curious about it. Don't fret; we've got your back. A period is short for menstruation, the time of the menstrual cycle during which women <u>bleed</u> . And just what is a menstrual cycle, exactly? Let's break this down!

<u>Hormones</u> rule your menstrual cycle and direct all the bodily functions that occur during this time. The first day of your period marks the beginning of each new cycle, which may last for as long as a week. Various hormones (estradiol, luteinizing, and follicle-stimulating hormones) rise and work together to wake up the ovaries during the first two weeks.

Now things get interesting. Around day 14 of your menstrual cycle, these hormones drop, and guess what? The ovaries send an <u>egg</u> down to the uterus. This is the time when the hormone progesterone starts to kick in. Its job is to thicken the lining of your uterus, just in case an egg gets fertilized by a sperm. The uterus would be all set to nourish the fertilized egg.

If no <u>fertilization</u> occurs, progesterone falls off, and the uterus sheds its lining. This shedding causes your period, and the blood contains the remnants of the old, unused uterine lining, and the whole process starts again.

It's essential to understand your menstrual cycle patterns and be prepared for your period by having access to pads, tampons, or menstrual cups because it could start unexpectedly. Also, it's not uncommon to experience stomach <u>cramps</u> , bloating, or mood swings during menstruation. Don't worry; there are many ways to manage the pain and discomfort that come with your period.

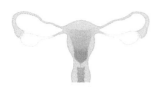

What's the Average Age to Start Your Period?

intimate	develops	experience	dreading	menstruation

It was a typical day in the small town of Maple Valley. The sun was shining, and birds were singing, but it was time for a very important conversation-one that mom had been dreading since her daughters started getting older.

Mom gathered her two girls, Jill and Sarah, into the living room and took a deep breath before beginning to talk about what many young women experience at some point in their lives: starting their period.

The girls looked up with wide eyes as Mom explained what happens during menstruation and why taking care of your body is essential when this natural process begins. She shared stories from when she first got her period, emphasizing how scary yet exciting it can be. Then she asked them if they had any questions about the topic or felt uncomfortable talking about it; thankfully, both girls seemed surprisingly comfortable discussing such an intimate subject!

Next, Mom wanted to ensure they knew exactly when they should expect such changes in their bodies, which vary greatly depending on age. After doing some research together online (and taking breaks for snacks!), they discovered that most girls start having periods between ages 10 and 15; however, there is no exact average age because everyone's body develops differently over time!

Jill and Sarah left the conversation feeling confident that they now knew enough information to recognize when these changes might occur within each of them individually-significantly, if Mom or Dad could help answer any other questions along the way!

Extra Credit: What does the word menstruation means?

[Student worksheet has a 5 line writing exercise here.]

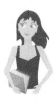

How Long Does a Normal Period Last

Are you wondering how long your period will last and how often it will come? Well, let me explain it to you in more detail!

First of all, your period usually lasts between two and seven days. But don't worry if it lasts a little longer or shorter than that, because everyone's body is different. Typically, the first two to three days are the heaviest, and then it gradually becomes lighter from there. So make sure to always have some pads or tampons with you, just in case!

Now, let's talk about how often you will get your period. This can be a bit tricky because your cycle might not be the same length every month. While the average cycle length is 28 days, it can actually range from 21 to 35 days. Sometimes, your period might come a little earlier or later than expected. But don't worry; this is totally normal!

In fact, your period will probably be unpredictable and irregular for the first few months. This is because your body is still adjusting to the changes happening inside of it. But after a while, you will be able to notice a pattern and figure out when your next period is coming.

One great way to track your period is by using a period-tracking app. There are lots of free ones available, which can help you track when your period is expected to arrive. This can also help you plan ahead and ensure you always have the necessary supplies.

So there you have it! Your period usually lasts between two and seven days, and might come at different times every month. But don't worry; it's all a normal part of growing up. And remember, if you ever have any questions or concerns, don't be afraid to talk to your doctor or another trusted adult.

1. Typically, your period may last anywhere from ___ to ___ days.
- a. two, seven
- b. three, six

2. The first two to three days of your menstruation are the ___.
- a. lightest
- b. heaviest

3. The typical length of a menstrual cycle is ___ days.
- a. 28
- b. 32

4. For the first few months, you may experience unpredictable and ___ bleeding.
- a. irregular
- b. regular

5. Your menstrual cycle may not occur at the same time each ___.
- a. month
- b. day

6. You'll eventually detect a ___ and figure out when your next period is due.
- a. symptoms
- b. pattern

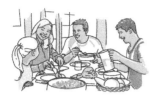

First Period Symptoms

It was a typical Sunday afternoon in the Robinson household. Dad, Mom, and their daughter Alice were all sitting around the kitchen table discussing school and upcoming plans for the week.

Suddenly, Dad cleared his throat and looked at Alice with an expression of seriousness that caught her by surprise. He said, "Alice, your mom has already had a chat with you about periods, but I wanted to make sure you know that if there's ever anything uncomfortable or embarrassing that you want to talk about—no matter what it is —I'm here for you too."

Alice shifted uncomfortably in her chair as she tried to guess where this conversation was going. The word "period" made her feel embarrassed; she knew what they meant but still felt like she didn't have enough information on them yet.

Dad noticed her discomfort, so he softened his tone as he continued talking. "I know this can be a confusing topic, so let me explain some of the things you may experience before getting your first period. You might notice changes in mood or energy levels—feeling tired more often than usual or maybe being extra emotional—these are all normal signs."

He went on to list other symptoms such as bloating and cramps from increased hormone levels, changes in skin texture due to oil production, and spotting caused by shedding of the uterine lining during the menstrual cycle preparation stages.

By now, Alice felt much more comfortable listening in on this important lesson from Dad. She thanked him for taking time out of his day to help educate her on something that could otherwise feel awkward or embarrassing to discuss openly with parents, especially dads.

1. Before receiving your period, you might experience _____ or energy changes.

    a. mood

    b. fever

2. Who educated Alice on first-period symptoms in this story?

    a. Dad

    b. Mom

3. Period symptoms such as _____ and _____ are caused by an increase in hormone levels.

    a. blemishes, chills

    b. bloating, cramping

4. During menstrual cycle preparation, the lining of the uterus sheds, causing ___.

    a. spotting

    b. light bruising

5. Where did this story take place?

    a. at the kitchen table

    b. in Alice's bedroom

6. Early menstruation signs of increased oil production causes ___ texture changes.

    a. hair

    b. skin

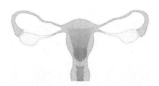

Reproductive Health Words You Should Know

Match the clues to the words. Need help? Try Google.

			⁸I							³G	
	⁷H	Y	M	E	N					E	
			M		⁶H	O	R	M	O	N	E	S
⁴F	E	T	U	S						I	
I			N							T	
B	²G	E	S	T	A	T	I	O	N	A	
R			S							L	
O	¹G	Y	N	E	C	O	L	O	G	I	S	T
I			S								
D			T								
			E								
			M								

Across

1. A doctor who specializes in health care for the vulva, vagina, uterus, ovaries, and breasts.
2. The period of time when a fetus is developing in the womb.
4. Develops from the embryo at 10 weeks of pregnancy and receives nourishment through the placenta.
6. Chemicals that cause changes in our bodies and brains.
7. A thin, fleshy piece of tissue that stretches across part of the opening to the vagina.

Down

3. External sex and reproductive organs, like the the vulva, penis, and scrotum.
4. A benign tumor that grows on the walls of the uterus.
8. The body's natural protection against infection and disease.

IMMUNE SYSTEM
GYNECOLOGIST   HYMEN
FIBROID   HORMONES
GENITALS   FETUS
GESTATION

Breast Pain

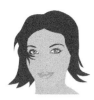

Chole was a 10th-grade girl who loved playing soccer. She had been playing on the girls' team since 8th grade and was one of the best players. However, Chole was worried about a problem that she had been having lately. She was experiencing breast pain, which was beginning to affect her game on the field. To make matters worse, her aunt passed away from breast cancer a few years ago, and she was scared it could happen to her.

Chole decided to go to her team's sports medicine doctor, Dr. McPherson. Dr. McPherson had been the team's doctor for years, and Chole had known her since the 4th grade. Dr. McPherson was a kind older lady who always had a smile on her face. Chole knew that she could trust her with her worries and concerns.

Dr. McPherson listened intently as Chole explained her symptoms and concerns about breast cancer. She reassured Chole that breast pain was common for many women, especially around the time of their menstrual cycle. She explained that the pain could be caused by a decrease in hormones and suggested some tips and tricks to ease the pain. Dr. McPherson suggested that Chole cut back on salt, sugar, caffeine, and dairy, as these could be contributing factors. She also recommended that Chole wear a supportive bra to help reduce the pain.

Dr. McPherson further explained that breast pain, although uncomfortable, is rarely linked to breast cancer. Dr. Johnson continued to explain the different types of breast pain. She learned that there are two main types: cyclic breast pain and noncyclic breast pain. Cyclic breast pain is linked to menstrual periods; with noncyclic breast pain, the breasts themselves could be the source of the pain. Or, it could be coming from somewhere else, like nearby muscles or joints, and could be felt in the breast. She encouraged Chole to perform regular self-examinations and to see her if she noticed any unusual changes.

As Chole left Dr. McPherson, she felt relieved and hopeful. She knew that breast pain could be uncomfortable, but it wasn't something to be worried about. She was grateful to Dr. McPherson for her guidance and kindness. Chole went back to playing soccer with renewed energy and confidence. She knew she could count on Dr. McPherson for her health concerns, giving her peace of mind.

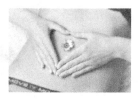

Managing a Heavy Period

For many of us, the thought of dealing with a heavy period can be overwhelming and frustrating. It's natural to worry about whether we'll leak through our tampon or pad, or if we'll even make it through the day without constant trips to the restroom. While some women experience lighter periods, others are prone to heavier cycles, known as menorrhagia.

But the question on most women's minds is: Is it normal to have heavy periods? The answer is not as simple, as everybody is different, and depending on who you ask, you might hear them say that there is no "normal" period. However, suppose you're experiencing bleeding that lasts longer than seven days, soaking through more than one pad or tampon every hour, passing blood clots larger than a quarter, or experiencing fatigue, weakness, or shortness of breath. In that case, your heavy period may be considered abnormal.

So, what qualifies as "heavy menstrual bleeding"? Generally speaking, women lose around 30–70 milliliters (mL) of menstrual blood during their periods. But when you're losing significantly more than that, it warrants concern. Losing 80 mL or more of blood per cycle or having a menstrual cycle that lasts longer than seven days are both signs of menorrhagia.

What are the symptoms of menorrhagia? Heavy menstrual bleeding is associated with numerous side effects, including fatigue, weakness, headaches, nausea, and mood changes. Women with menorrhagia may also experience stomach cramps, lower back pain, pain during intercourse, and frequent urination.

So, how can you manage heavy periods and avoid feeling overwhelmed? First, keep track of your menstrual cycle with a period tracker app, marking down when your period starts and ends and how much blood you lose each day. This will give you a clear idea of whether your bleeding exceeds the average loss of 30–70 mL per cycle. Secondly, consider using menstrual products such as period underwear, which can hold up to two tampons worth of menstrual blood, or menstrual cups, which can hold more fluid and be worn for up to 12 hours.

Aside from wearable products, medical management methods can also help. It's always best to consult your doctor to discuss these options and see which would work best for you.

Lastly, what causes heavy periods? While there is no exact cause of menorrhagia, it can be attributed to various factors such as hormonal imbalances and underlying medical conditions like thyroid dysfunction, uterine fibroids, and polyps. However, these factors may not apply to everyone, and you may be experiencing heavy periods due to other reasons like stress, poor nutrition, and lifestyle habits.

In conclusion, menorrhagia is a common issue that many women face, but there are numerous ways to manage and overcome it. By keeping track of your menstrual cycle, using wearable products, consulting with your doctor, and leading a healthy lifestyle, you can alleviate the burden of a heavy period and enjoy a more comfortable and relaxed monthly cycle. Remember that you can take care of your menstrual cycle and trust that your body can manage even the most difficult of periods without compromising your health or happiness.

1. Period blood loss averages between ___ and 70 mL for most women.

    a. 45

    b. 30

2. Heavily bleeding periods are also known as _____.

    a. menorrhagia

    b. mensuration

3. _____, poor nutrition, and unhealthy habits are all possible causes of your heavy periods.

    a. Stress

    b. Mood

4. Menorrhagia is diagnosed when a woman loses ____ mL or more of blood per cycle or has a _____-day cycle.

    a. 80, seven

    b. 30, six

Period Cramps

muscle	stretching	heating	laughing	experiencing

"Come on, sweetie," Dr. Miller said gently to the young girl sitting before him. Dr. Miller has been the young girl's doctor since she was a baby, so she knew the doctor very well. Dr. Miller said, "I know this isn't easy to talk about, but I'm here to help you."

The girl looked up at him nervously; her hands were clasped tightly together, and her eyes welled with tears. She had been experiencing period cramps for some time now, but she didn't feel comfortable going to her parents or friends for help.

Dr. Miller smiled kindly at the girl before continuing his advice: "Period cramps can be tough; they're like any other kind of cramp, where a muscle contracts too hard or too fast and makes it difficult for your body to move around easily." He paused as he saw understanding slowly dawning in the girls' expression before continuing: "But there are things that you can do!" "A heating pad is always a good idea if you have one; it helps soothe those muscles that are contracting too quickly."

He then went on to explain how exercise could also be beneficial; gentle movements such as walking or stretching would help loosen up your muscles and reduce pain levels. Then he added something that made the young girl smile: "And don't forget that even though it may not seem like it right now, laughing is actually an effective way of managing pain!" "So make sure you take some time out from all this discomforting stuff and find something funny!"

As he finished speaking, Dr. Miller's face softened into a warm smile; his words had done their job of calming down the troubled teen before him. The young girl returned his smile gratefully before hugging him goodbye and leaving with newfound confidence in tackling her period cramps head-on!

Extra Credit: List 4 things that can help ease cramps. Use Google to research your answer if needed.

[Student worksheet has a 5 line writing exercise here.]

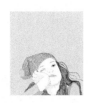

Phases of the Menstrual Cycle

Menstruation is a normal biological process that occurs in females between puberty and menopause . The menstrual cycle is divided into four phases, each with unique characteristics and functions: the follicular phase, ovulation, luteal phase, and menstruation.

Firstly, the follicular phase is the first phase of the menstrual cycle. It starts on the first day (1-14) of menstruation and lasts for approximately two weeks. During this phase, the follicles in the ovary begin to mature and produce estrogen. The lining of the uterus also begins to thicken in preparation for a potential pregnancy. As the follicular phase progresses, one follicle becomes dominant and continues to grow, while the others shrink and die off.

The second phase of the menstrual cycle is ovulation. If you have a 28 day cycle, this phase occurs around day 14 of the menstrual cycle and lasts for about 24 to 48 hours. During ovulation, the dominant follicle releases an egg into the fallopian tube. The egg travels through the tube towards the uterus and can be fertilized by sperm during this journey. If the egg is not fertilized, it should disintegrate within 24 hours of its release.

Following ovulation is the luteal phase, days 15-28. During this phase, the ruptured follicle transforms into the corpus luteum, which produces progesterone. Progesterone helps thicken and prepare the uterus for the potential implantation of a fertilized egg. If fertilization does not occur, the corpus luteum disintegrates, causing a drop in progesterone levels.

Lastly, menstruation is the phase that marks the end of the menstrual cycle. It typically lasts for 3-7 days, and during this phase, the thickened lining of the uterus sheds , and blood and other materials exit the body through the vagina. This process is the beginning of a new menstrual cycle.

It is important to note that the length and characteristics of the menstrual cycle can vary from person to person. Certain factors like stress, illness, and weight changes can also affect the menstrual cycle.

In conclusion, the menstrual cycle is a normal biological process that occurs in females. It consists of four phases, each with unique characteristics and functions: the follicular phase, ovulation, the luteal phase, and menstruation. Understanding the menstrual cycle can help females track their menstrual cycle, monitor their health, and make informed decisions about their reproductive health.

Period Cycle Fill-in-Blanks

The lining of the uterus thickens monthly from puberty to menopause in preparation for potential pregnancy. Because of this, a fertilized egg can successfully implant in the uterus and you can get pregnant.

In a nutshell, if an egg is not implanted, the thicker tissue is shed by the body. Periods involve the monthly outflow of blood and tissue through the vagina.

The menstrual cycle is a monthly biological process that consists of several phases. Menstrual periods typically last between 21 and 40 days, while the average length is closer to 28 days.

Your cycle contains several phases that serve distinct functions and are followed by corresponding signs and symptoms.

_____

During this exercise, you will fill in the blanks with the correct word to match the definitions or clues.

hormonal	important	luteal	conception	ovulation
menstrual	bleeding	increase	follicular	cycle

1. Menstruation is an important part of life for teenage girls.

2. The average menstrual cycle usually lasts 28 days, though this can vary from person to person.

3. During a 28-day cycle, hormonal changes occur, which lead to ovulation, menstruation, and other bodily changes.

4. For teenagers, it's particularly helpful to understand menstrual cycle changes so they can better prepare themselves for what may come.

5. The first stage of the menstrual cycle is the follicular phase, where hormones are released that cause the egg in the ovary to mature.

6. The ovulation phase is when a mature egg is released from the ovary into the fallopian tube and is ready for fertilization if sperm are present.

7. The third stage of the menstrual cycle is called the luteal phase.

8. During the luteal phase, hormone levels increase to maintain a pregnancy should conception occur.

9. If no conception occurs, then the final stage begins menstruation.

10. During menstruation, eggs, and uterine lining shed, resulting in bleeding that typically lasts 3-7 days before starting over again with a new cycle beginning with the follicular phase.

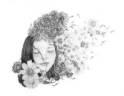

When Do Most Girls Get Their Period

In this activity, you'll see grammatical *errors*. Correct all the grammar mistakes you see.

> There are **7** mistakes in this passage. 1 capital missing. 2 unnecessary capitals. 4 incorrectly spelled words.

~~once~~ **Once** upon a time, a young girl named Sophie had many questions about growing up. One day she asked her mom, "Mom, when do most girls get their period?"

Her mom smiled and said, "Most girls get their period for the first ~~tame~~ **time** around age 12, but it can happen earlier or later. Before your period starts, you might notice some changes ~~In~~ **in** your ~~budy,~~ **body,** like breast growth or acne, and you might feel moody."

Sophie was happy to have her questions answered as she thought about what it would be like when her own period came. Her mom added that it could be different each month, with lighter or heavier bleeding and sometimes cramps or other PMS symptoms like headaches.

She said it's essential to take care of Sophie's body - ~~eatang~~ **eating** right, getting enough sleep, and exercising, and ~~Talking~~ **talking** to an adult she trusts about any questions she has.

"I guess I ~~hive~~ **have** some things to look forward to," Sophie said with a smile.

First Visit to the Gynecologist

Monica was a shy 14-year-old girl. She had only ever been to her pediatrician and dentist, and the thought of visiting a gynecologist made her anxious. Her mom had been encouraging her to see one, especially since her menstrual cycle had started a few months ago.

She felt uneasy about the visit, not knowing what to expect. As she stepped into the gynecologist's office, she was taken aback by the sterile and unfamiliar surroundings, unlike her pediatrician's warm and friendly office.

Her heart was pounding, and her palms were sweaty as she waited for her turn to see the doctor. Her mind was swirling with questions. What would the doctor ask her? Would it hurt? Would it be embarrassing? All those thoughts made her feel vulnerable and uncomfortable.

As she sat in the consulting room, the gynecologist, Dr. Garcia, walked in. She had a warm and friendly smile that calmed Monica's nerves. Dr. Garcia asked about Monica's menstrual cycle, lifestyle and health habits, family health history, and whether she is sexually active. She answered all her questions about menstrual hygiene, sexual health, and reproductive health.

She explained, in detail, the importance of seeing a gynecologist at least once a year for early detection and prevention of any health issues. Dr. Garcia also taught Monica the importance of carrying herself with self-respect and dignity, even when confronted with obstacles in her life.

Monica was relieved that the consultation wasn't as frightening as she thought it would be. She felt a sense of empowerment and confidence that only came from taking charge of her body and health.

As Monica headed out of the clinic, she found herself walking taller and more assured than before. She knew that taking care of her body was an important part of growing up to become a healthy and responsible adult. She had learned that regular check-ups were a vital part of this and she felt optimistic and confident about her overall health.

Indeed, Monica's first visit to a gynecologist was a turning point in her life, and one that she would always look back on with gratitude. She no longer feared visiting a gynecologist, knowing that her health and well-being were more important.

Side Note: Between the ages of 13 and 15, doctors advise young women to get their first gynecological exam. Most girls have already started puberty by then, so it's an excellent time to ensure everything is growing normally.

Breast and pelvic exams are usually unnecessary for young women until they reach the age of 21. However, a pelvic exam may be performed if the doctor or nurse suspects something is wrong (or if you are experiencing symptoms such as abnormally heavy bleeding, missed periods, vaginal sores or itchiness, discharge, or other problems). Your doctor may perform a breast or pelvic examination if you have a family history of disease, especially if the disease is reproductive-related.

1. Young women under _____ rarely need breast and pelvic exams.
   a. 30
   b. 21

2. The importance of seeing a gynecologist at least _____ a year for early detection and prevention of health disorders.
   a. once
   b. twice

3. Doctors recommend a first gynecological exam for girls between _____ and _____.
   a. 16, 18
   b. 13, 15

4. Your doctor may examine your _____ or _____ if you have a family history of disease.
   a. breasts, pelvis
   b. bleeding, skin

Can I Skip My Period?

menopause	summer	remedies	nature	methods

Kim was so excited about her upcoming sweet sixteen pool party. She had been planning it all summer , from the decorations to the perfect playlist. But now that the day was almost here, she had a problem-she didn't want to start her period on her birthday!

She decided to take matters into her own hands and asked around for advice on how to skip it. Her friends told her about a few different methods they had heard about on social media, but Kim wasn't sure if they were safe or reliable, so she chose not to try them out.

She called up her grandmother, a wise woman in her seventies who was known for having natural remedies for any ailment. Unfortunately, Kim didn't get the response she hoped for. Granny told Kim that certain forms of hormonal birth control could enable a woman to skip her period. However, besides that, it wasn't safe or proven to stop your period outside of pregnancy or menopause . Granny wasn't too keen on this idea and again advised against it: "Kim, it is not safe or healthy for you at your age," Granny said firmly but kindly. "Let nature take its course." Granny then warned Kim against taking medical advice from social media and her friends as well.

Kim reluctantly accepted this advice but still felt disappointed that she wouldn't have a "perfect" birthday without being on her period. As days passed leading up to the party, though, something strange happened-miraculously enough, by some divine intervention perhaps, when it came time for Kim's birthday party: there was no sign of Aunt Flo! It seemed like nature had taken its own course after all-just as Granny said it would!

The rest of the night went off without a hitch, and everyone enjoyed themselves tremendously! When Kim thanked Granny later that week over a Skype call (since Granny didn't make it to her party), Granny just winked with a smile and said, "Grandmother knows best!"

Extra Credit: 1) What did Kim's Granny advise her about skipping her period? 2) What does the word menopause mean? Use Google to research your answer if needed.

[Student worksheet has a 3 line writing exercise here.]

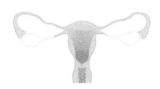

Reproductive Health Words You Should Know

Match the clues to the words. Need help? Try Google.

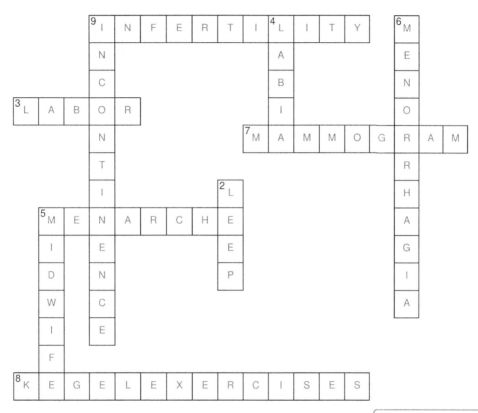

Across

3. The process of childbirth.
5. The first time a person gets their period.
7. A breast/chest cancer screening that takes x-rays of the breasts/chest tissue to find lumps.
8. The tightening and releasing of the muscles that stop urination in order to prevent and improve urinary incontinence.
9. The inability to become pregnant or to cause a pregnancy.

Down

2. A treatment that prevents cervical cancer.
4. The lips of the vulva.
5. A health care provider who is trained to assist in childbirth.
6. Menstrual bleeding that's heavier or longer lasting than usual.
9. Being unable to control urination or bowel movements.

LABOR LABIA INFERTILITY
MAMMOGRAM
MENORRHAGIA MIDWIFE
INCONTINENCE LEEP
MENARCHE KEGEL
EXERCISES

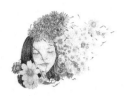

Dark Red Period Blood

In this activity, you'll see grammatical *errors*. Correct all the grammar mistakes you see.

There are **9** mistakes in this passage. 1 capital missing. 2 unnecessary capitals. 6 incorrectly spelled words.

Carla was ~~fealing~~ **feeling** a bit anxious. She had just started her period, and the blood on her pad wasn't red like she expected. Instead, it was black. ~~she~~ **She** was a nervous wreck-after all, something must have gone wrong if the color of her menstrual ~~bloud~~ **blood** looked so strange!

She decided to ask someone who would know more than her: Aunt Kelly, who is a nurse by profession. Carla nervously explained what happened and asked why this could be happening to her body.

Aunt Kelly calmly replied that it's normal for period blood to sometimes ~~Be~~ **be** dark brown or even black at the beginning or end of your cycle. When flow is slow during these ~~tames,~~ **times,** old blood can get exposed to oxygen, which causes iron in the blood cells to oxidize and become darker. But she added that if menstrual bleeding stays black throughout an ~~Entire~~ **entire** cycle, there may be cause for concern! She told Carla not to hesitate to tell her mom and contact a healthcare provider should anything else ~~seam~~ **seem** off with regard to menstruation health from that point forward; better safe than sorry!

Carla felt relieved after hearing Aunt Kelly's explanation but also empowered knowing she now had all the necessary ~~informatoin~~ **information** about what happens when you start your period, including having insight into why one might experience different colors of menstrual ~~floid~~ **fluid** occasionally over time!

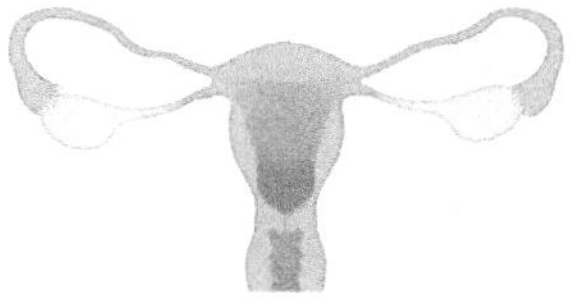

ANSWER SHEET

Reproductive Health Words You Should Know

Match the clues to the words. Need help? Try Google.

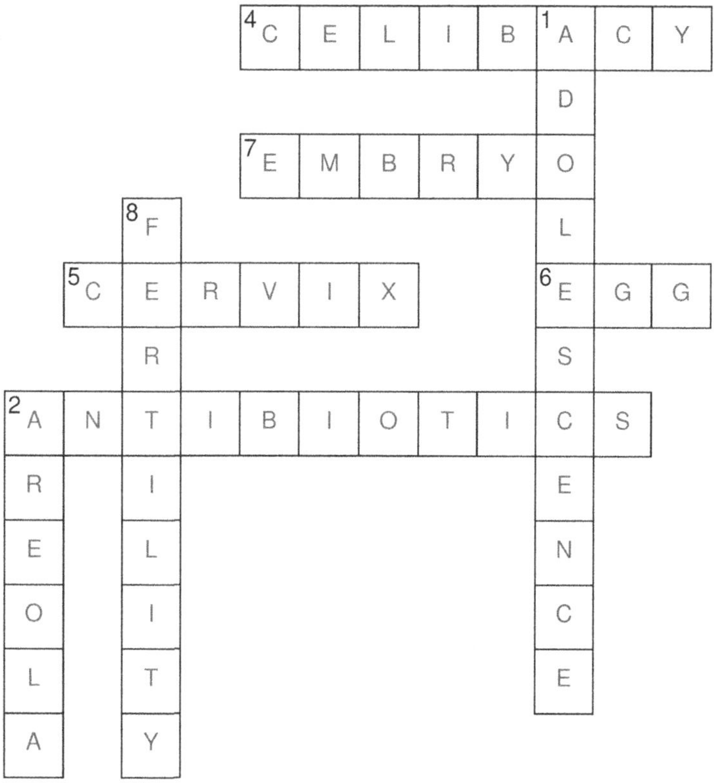

Across

2. Medicines that are used to cure infections caused by bacteria.
4. Not having sex.
5. The narrow, lower part of the uterus, with a small opening connecting the uterus to the vagina.
6. The reproductive cell stored in the ovaries and released during ovulation.
7. The organism that develops from a pre-embryo during the second month of pregnancy.

Down

1. The period of physical and emotional change between the beginning of puberty and early adulthood.
2. The dark area surrounding the nipple.
8. The ability to have children or cause a pregnancy.

EMBRYO AREOLA
ADOLESCENCE CERVIX
FERTILITY ANTIBIOTICS
EGG CELIBACY

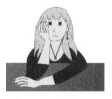

What happens during PMS?

Today, we will talk about something that affects almost every woman at some point in her life: PMS or Premenstrual Syndrome. PMS is a complex group of symptoms that affect women during the luteal phase of their menstrual cycle, which is the period between ovulation and menstruation.

PMS is a collection of physical and emotional symptoms that occur in the week leading up to your period. Hormonal fluctuations in your body cause it as your ovaries prepare to release an egg. These hormonal changes can affect the levels of serotonin, a chemical in the brain that regulates mood, appetite, and sleep.

So, what are the most common symptoms of PMS? Well, there are a few, and they can range from mild bloating and mood swings to severe cramping and headaches. Some of the most common PMS symptoms include:

1. Mood swings
2. Breast tenderness
3. Bloating
4. Acne breakouts
5. Fatigue
6. Headaches
7. Cravings
8. Insomnia
9. Irritability and anxiety

If you're experiencing any of these symptoms, don't worry; you can do several things to help ease them. Here are some tips:

1. Exercise regularly
2. Reduce your salt and sugar intake
3. Eat a balanced diet rich in vitamins, minerals, and healthy fats and drink plenty of water
4. Take painkillers, such as ibuprofen or acetaminophen, for pain relief
5. Use heat therapy for abdominal cramps, such as a hot water bottle or warm towel
6. Practice relaxation techniques, such as yoga, meditation, or deep breathing

But why do we experience PMS, you may ask? Well, the exact cause of PMS isn't known yet, but medical researchers think it has something to do with the changes in hormones during the menstrual cycle. Hormones such as estrogen and progesterone help regulate our menstrual cycle and influence our mood, energy levels, and physical health. When there's an imbalance of these hormones during the luteal phase, it can lead to the various symptoms of PMS.

To summarize, PMS is a group of symptoms that can affect women during the luteal phase of their menstrual cycle. Symptoms can range from mild to severe. While the exact cause isn't known, you can do things to ease PMS symptoms, such as exercise and eating a balanced diet. Remember, it's all part of being a woman, and with these tips, you'll be able to manage your PMS symptoms without letting them interfere with your daily life.

1. PMS is characterized by a number of _____ and _____ symptoms.

    a. monthly cycles. bleeding

    b. physical, emotional

2. What does the acronym PMS mean?

    a. Premenstrual Syndrome

    b. Premedical Symptoms

3. Serotonin is a _____ in the brain that affects mood, hunger, and sleep.

    a. chemical

    b. tissue

4. _____ and progesterone are two hormones that help control our monthly cycle.

    a. Melatonin

    b. Estrogen

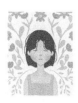

2 Periods in One Month

| hormones | cycles | irregular | uterine | periods |

Tina was a junior in high school and had been experiencing something strange with her periods . She would have them twice in the same month, which seemed to be happening more often. She knew that wasn't normal, so one day, she decided to go talk to the nurse at her school about it.

When she arrived, she felt relieved that someone else might finally understand what was going on. As soon as they started talking, the nurse explained how having menstrual cycles 21 days apart could lead to having two periods per month; however, this could also indicate other health issues, such as ovarian cysts, endometriosis, uterine fibroids, pelvic inflammatory disease, and cervical neoplasia. Tina thought back over the past few months, trying to remember if there had been any other signs of anything being wrong, but nothing had come up for her until now.

The nurse told Tina not to worry too much yet but told her to see a doctor in case something important was going on under all those hormones and bleeding cycles. With a smile of understanding, Tina thanked the nurse for her time and felt much better about her situation.

Tina made an appointment with her doctor right away because, although irregular bleeding can sometimes be normal during puberty, it's essential not to take any risks when it comes to your body's health!

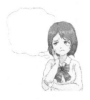

Why Is My Period Late?

pregnancy	diet	research	overnight	anxious

Samantha had been feeling off for weeks. She was tired, her stomach hurt constantly, and she felt anxious all the time. But now that it was almost June, another thing had started to bother her: why was her period late? As Samantha tried to figure out what could be causing this, she decided it was best to talk to someone about it.

She knew one person who would know how to handle the situation: her cool older sister, Lily. Lily always seemed so wise beyond her years, and Samantha trusted her opinion more than anyone else's. So when they were alone in their room that night, Samantha nervously asked, "Why is my period late?"

Lily immediately smiled reassuringly and pulled out a notebook from underneath her bed. Inside were pages upon pages of notes from medical journals she read as part of research projects for school (she wanted to be a doctor someday). After explaining some possible causes like stress, diet change, or being under the weather-which made sense given how things had been going lately-she then mentioned pregnancy as an unlikely but still potential cause.

Samantha thanked Lily for the new information before getting ready for bed with new knowledge in hand and hope in her heart; everything would ultimately work itself out just fine! Samantha now realizes that these problems won't go away overnight , and that's okay, too!

Extra Credit: What are irregular periods?

[Student worksheet has a 5 line writing exercise here.]

Vaginal Discharge

Vaginal discharge, as uncomfortable and embarrassing as it may seem, is an entirely normal and healthy process that happens to all girls and women with vaginas. It's a fluid that comes from the vagina and helps clean and moisturize it while also protecting against infections.

Some of you may have noticed this on the toilet paper when you wipe or in your underwear. That's because it's perfectly normal for the quantity, texture, and color of the discharge to change throughout the month, depending on your menstrual cycle. However, some changes in discharge can signal a problem, indicating that it's time to consult your doctor.

Normal vaginal discharge can vary in color, texture, and amount between different individuals, depending on several factors such as age, menstrual cycle, pregnancy, or even stress levels. However, it's essential to identify what's usual for your body to notice when something is out of the ordinary and seek medical advice if necessary.

Generally speaking, normal vaginal discharge should be clear, white, or off-white in color, and it shouldn't smell unpleasant, burn, itch, or cause irritation. It's also common for some girls to have a more substantial amount of vaginal discharge than others, which might require wearing a pantyliner to keep their underwear dry. On the other hand, some girls do not have much discharge at all, which can also be entirely normal.

When it comes to the texture of the discharge, it can vary from thin, sticky, and elastic to a thick, gooey consistency, depending on the menstrual cycle phase. For instance, the discharge can become more stretchy and slippery during ovulation, allowing the sperm to swim more easily. Toward the end of the menstrual cycle, the discharge can become slightly thicker and stickier to form a plug that prevents infection from entering the cervix.

However, some changes in the discharge may indicate a problem that requires medical attention. For instance, if the discharge is yellow or green, has a strong smell, appears curdled or cottage cheese-like, or comes with itching, burning, or pain, it might indicate an infection. Yeast (candidiasis), bacteria (bacterial vaginosis), or sexually transmitted infections (STIs) like chlamydia or gonorrhea are some of the most common causes of vaginal infections.

In conclusion, vaginal discharge is a natural and normal process that varies from person to person and throughout the menstrual cycle. It's essential to know what's typical for your body to identify any changes that might signal an infection, especially if they are accompanied by discomfort or odor. If you suspect an infection, don't hesitate to speak to your parent(s) or a healthcare provider, who can diagnose and treat the problem if necessary. Remember, taking care of your vaginal health is essential to maintaining overall well-being, and it starts with awareness and education.

1. Vaginal discharge should be clear, white, or off-white, and _____.

    a. odorless

    b. slight smell

2. Depending on the menstrual cycle phase, the discharge might be thin, sticky, elastic, or _____ and gooey.

    a. thick

    b. bloody

3. At the end of the menstrual cycle, the discharge might thicken and cling to the _____, preventing infection.

    a. cervix

    b. vagina

4. Some girls need a _____ to keep their underwear dry because they have more vaginal discharge than others.

    a. tampon

    b. pantyliner

5. If the discharge is yellow or green, smells unpleasant, looks curdled or cottage cheese-like, itches, burns, or hurts, it may be an _____.

    a. infection

    b. pregnancy

6. Vaginal infections are often caused by _____, bacteria, or STIs like chlamydia or gonorrhea.

    a. birth control

    b. yeast

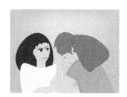

Yeast Infection

Trina was working the Friday evening shift at the local movie theatre. She had been feeling discomfort and itching around her vagina for a few days but hadn't thought much about it until that night. On her break, Trina went to the bathroom and noticed that she was red, and there appeared to be some irritation on her skin. She immediately called her best friend Lisa in a panic, asking, "How can I tell if I have a yeast infection?"

Lisa cracked an inappropriate joke instead of answering: "Why did the rich woman sell yeast? Then Lisa giggled and said, "To raise some dough." Trina wasn't amused by this joke (not even finding it remotely funny). Lisa then told Trina that she wasn't sure because she never had one before and that she should seek medical advice as soon as possible so they could diagnose her correctly.

Trina couldn't get an appointment with her primary physician until Monday, so instead, she went to the weekend clinic where her mom worked for help on Saturday morning. When she arrived, Trina told them what had been going on. After noting down all of her symptoms and collecting a urine sample, the doctor informed Trina that although the itching suggested it could be a yeast infection, luckily for her, it wasn't one! Instead, he concluded that it was likely due to an allergic reaction from recently using new soap or detergent, which had caused the irritation. Tina then remembered that she was using this new body wash she received last month as a Christmas gift.

The doctor also educated Trina further; he advised that yeast infections can cause a vaginal discharge that resembles cottage cheese and is thick and white. The discharge can be watery and often smell-less. He continued and said that, usually, to check for inflammation and discharge; most doctors will perform a pelvic exam. With a cotton swab, a doctor can collect a sample of the discharge coming from the patient's vagina. From there, the sample will be examined under a microscope to determine whether the patient has a yeast infection. He added that the pelvic exam wasn't necessary in her case because she had no other symptoms. And in the future, he said, use a mild, unscented soap or plain water. Using a new body wash, especially one with fragrance, can disturb the pH of your vagina and cause irritation or a yeast infection.

Trina thanked the doctor for his help and left after hearing this news. She has learned her lesson and will take extra precautions to maintain her personal hygiene in the future to avoid similar incidents.

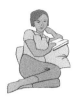

Different Menstrual Products

Sanitary Pads

Sanitary pads, or napkins, are the most commonly used menstrual product. They are attached to the inside of the woman's underwear and work by absorbing menstrual blood through layers of absorbent material like rayon , cotton, and plastic. Over the decades, the design of pads has evolved to become much more absorbent and comfortable, with a wide range available to suit different flows.

Tampons

Tampons are a popular option, which absorbs menstrual blood internally through vaginal insertion. Tampons can take practice, and not everyone finds them comfortable to use. They can be left in for about four hours, at which point they are removed by pulling gently on the string . Leaks are common with tampons, so an additional pantiliner may be required.

Menstrual Cups

In recent years, many people have given up the more traditional options of tampons and pads in favor of the menstrual cup. This small silicone or latex cup works by being folded and inserted internally, where it collects blood. They are a sustainable option since they can last for years with proper care. Menstrual cups take some time to get positioning right, but once the technique is mastered, leakages shouldn't be a problem, and they are comfortable and safe to use.

Menstrual Discs

The lesser-known menstrual disc, made of plastic or silicone, is also inserted into the vagina and rests on the base of the cervix. It can stay in for up to 12 hours and works by collecting blood in the disc. Menstrual discs can take some time to figure out how to use correctly, but they offer a sustainable and comfortable option.

Period Underwear

The latest newcomer to the period scene is period underwear. They look like regular underwear but have a special absorbent layer that prevents clothing leakage. As they are washable and reusable, they are one of the most sustainable options available. A good pair of period underwear will prevent odors, making them comfortable and discreet to the wearer.

It's essential for young women to experiment with different menstrual products and find the ones that are right for them. Each product has pros and cons, so choosing the one that suits their lifestyle and preferences is important. Changing them regularly and maintaining good hygiene to avoid infections is essential no matter what product they use. By knowing about the different menstrual products available, young women can take control of their menstrual cycle and lead a healthy, active life.

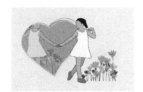

Body Image and Self-Esteem

She compared herself to the models and __influencers__ she saw on social media, feeling that she would never measure up.

The teasing and __catty__ remarks from her peers did not help.

Mrs. Bradley called her in for a chat, and soon Tiffany was pouring out her struggles with her body image and __low__ self-worth.

Mrs. Bradley then gave Tiffany practical advice on accepting herself for who she is rather than trying to keep up with societal __beauty__ standards.

She started to buy clothes that suited her body type while __experimenting__ with different hairstyles and accessories.

Her friends and even strangers __complimented__ her, and she started to get more positive attention, which boosted her morale.

The moral of the story is to be body positive and love yourself for who you are rather than putting yourself under immense pressure to fit in with __societal__ beauty standards.

Tiffany learned to appreciate her __unique__ attributes and embrace her identity. She felt empowered to be herself and began living life on her terms. The world can be a __dark__ place, but with a positive mindset and self-love, anything is possible.

Although a negative body image is a common struggle for many people, it can be improved by __incorporating__ some of these practical and actionable tips.

Practice Self-Care: Pamper yourself with small acts of self-care each day, such as taking a relaxing bath, getting enough __sleep__, and doing things you enjoy.

Start Your Day Positively: Begin your day positively by saying __affirmations__ and stating your intentions.

Spend time with people who make you feel good about yourself and avoid people that bring __negativity__ or criticism into your life.

Physical activity, such as cycling, running, or __yoga__, boosts mood and confidence as it interacts with endorphins.

Find Your Own Style: Dress up in clothing and colors that make you feel comfortable and __confident__.

Practice positive self-talk by replacing negative __thoughts__ with positive affirmations, as mentioned above.

Remember that social media is just curated content; what people show online is their highlight __reel__, not necessarily the reality.

Eat Healthily: Healthy eating can directly impact our health, __mood__, and self-esteem.

It will encourage positive self-talk, __boost__ your self-esteem, and improve your overall mood.

By incorporating these tips, you can build __healthier__ habits and create a positive outlook for your body and self-esteem.

Period Tracker

Cycle Day

1 2 3 4 5 6 7 8 9 10 11 12 13 14 15 16 17 18 19 20 21 22 23 24 25 26 27 28 29 30 31 32 33 34 35 36 37 38 39 40 41 42 43 44 45

Date: _____

Avg. Cycle Length: _____

Basal Body Temp: _____

Birth Control Method: _____

Took Birth Control: ☐ Yes ☐ No

Menstruating: ☐ Yes ☐ No

Ovulating: ☐ Yes ☐ No

Pregnant: ☐ Yes ☐ No

On Antibiotics: ☐ Yes ☐ No

Had Protected Sex: ☐ Yes ☐ No

Had Unprotected Sex: ☐ Yes ☐ No

Symptoms

☐ Spotting   ☐ Light Bleeding   ☐ Moderate Bleeding

☐ Heavy Bleeding   ☐ Acne/Breakout   ☐ Cramps

☐ Tender/Swollen Breasts ☐ Backache   ☐ Headache

☐ Joint Pain   ☐ Mood Swings   ☐ Anxiety/Depression

☐ Bloating   ☐ Constipation   ☐ Diarrhea

☐ Fatigue   ☐ Dizziness   ☐ Nausea/Vomiting

☐ Appetite Changes   ☐ Pelvic Pressure   ☐ Clots/Bloody Discharge

☐ Sticky Discharge   ☐ Creamy Discharge   ☐ Egg-White Discharge

☐ Other:

Notes

Period Tracker

Cycle Day

(circular day tracker: 1 2 3 4 5 6 7 8 9 10 11 12 13 14 15 16 17 18 19 20 21 22 23 24 25 26 27 28 29 30 31 32 33 34 35 36 37 38 39 40 41 42 43 44 45)

Date: _____

Avg. Cycle Length: _____

Basal Body Temp: _____

Birth Control Method: _____

Took Birth Control: ☐ Yes ☐ No

Menstruating: ☐ Yes ☐ No

Ovulating: ☐ Yes ☐ No

Pregnant: ☐ Yes ☐ No

On Antibiotics: ☐ Yes ☐ No

Had Protected Sex: ☐ Yes ☐ No

Had Unprotected Sex: ☐ Yes ☐ No

Symptoms

☐ Spotting	☐ Light Bleeding	☐ Moderate Bleeding
☐ Heavy Bleeding	☐ Acne/Breakout	☐ Cramps
☐ Tender/Swollen Breasts	☐ Backache	☐ Headache
☐ Joint Pain	☐ Mood Swings	☐ Anxiety/Depression
☐ Bloating	☐ Constipation	☐ Diarrhea
☐ Fatigue	☐ Dizziness	☐ Nausea/Vomiting
☐ Appetite Changes	☐ Pelvic Pressure	☐ Clots/Bloody Discharge
☐ Sticky Discharge	☐ Creamy Discharge	☐ Egg-White Discharge

☐ Other: _____

Notes

Period Tracker

Cycle Day

(circular dial numbered 1 through 45)

Date: _____

Avg. Cycle Length: _____

Basal Body Temp: _____

Birth Control Method: _____

Took Birth Control: ☐ Yes   ☐ No

Menstruating: ☐ Yes   ☐ No

Ovulating: ☐ Yes   ☐ No

Pregnant: ☐ Yes   ☐ No

On Antibiotics: ☐ Yes   ☐ No

Had Protected Sex: ☐ Yes   ☐ No

Had Unprotected Sex: ☐ Yes   ☐ No

Symptoms

☐ Spotting	☐ Light Bleeding	☐ Moderate Bleeding
☐ Heavy Bleeding	☐ Acne/Breakout	☐ Cramps
☐ Tender/Swollen Breasts	☐ Backache	☐ Headache
☐ Joint Pain	☐ Mood Swings	☐ Anxiety/Depression
☐ Bloating	☐ Constipation	☐ Diarrhea
☐ Fatigue	☐ Dizziness	☐ Nausea/Vomiting
☐ Appetite Changes	☐ Pelvic Pressure	☐ Clots/Bloody Discharge
☐ Sticky Discharge	☐ Creamy Discharge	☐ Egg-White Discharge

☐ Other: _____

Notes

Period Tracker

Cycle Day

(circular cycle day chart numbered 1 through 45)

Date: _____

Avg. Cycle Length: _____

Basal Body Temp: _____

Birth Control Method: _____

Took Birth Control:	☐ Yes	☐ No
Menstruating:	☐ Yes	☐ No
Ovulating:	☐ Yes	☐ No
Pregnant:	☐ Yes	☐ No
On Antibiotics:	☐ Yes	☐ No
Had Protected Sex:	☐ Yes	☐ No
Had Unprotected Sex:	☐ Yes	☐ No

Symptoms

☐ Spotting	☐ Light Bleeding	☐ Moderate Bleeding
☐ Heavy Bleeding	☐ Acne/Breakout	☐ Cramps
☐ Tender/Swollen Breasts	☐ Backache	☐ Headache
☐ Joint Pain	☐ Mood Swings	☐ Anxiety/Depression
☐ Bloating	☐ Constipation	☐ Diarrhea
☐ Fatigue	☐ Dizziness	☐ Nausea/Vomiting
☐ Appetite Changes	☐ Pelvic Pressure	☐ Clots/Bloody Discharge
☐ Sticky Discharge	☐ Creamy Discharge	☐ Egg-White Discharge

☐ Other: _____

Notes

Period Tracker

Cycle Day

(circular chart numbered 1 through 45)

Date: _____

Avg. Cycle Length: _____

Basal Body Temp: _____

Birth Control Method: _____

Took Birth Control: ☐ Yes ☐ No

Menstruating: ☐ Yes ☐ No

Ovulating: ☐ Yes ☐ No

Pregnant: ☐ Yes ☐ No

On Antibiotics: ☐ Yes ☐ No

Had Protected Sex: ☐ Yes ☐ No

Had Unprotected Sex: ☐ Yes ☐ No

Symptoms

☐ Spotting   ☐ Light Bleeding   ☐ Moderate Bleeding

☐ Heavy Bleeding   ☐ Acne/Breakout   ☐ Cramps

☐ Tender/Swollen Breasts ☐ Backache   ☐ Headache

☐ Joint Pain   ☐ Mood Swings   ☐ Anxiety/Depression

☐ Bloating   ☐ Constipation   ☐ Diarrhea

☐ Fatigue   ☐ Dizziness   ☐ Nausea/Vomiting

☐ Appetite Changes   ☐ Pelvic Pressure   ☐ Clots/Bloody Discharge

☐ Sticky Discharge   ☐ Creamy Discharge   ☐ Egg-White Discharge

☐ Other: _____

Notes

Period Tracker

Cycle Day

(circular chart with numbers 1 through 45 arranged around the center labeled "Cycle Day")

Date: _____

Avg. Cycle Length: _____

Basal Body Temp: _____

Birth Control Method: _____

Took Birth Control: ☐ Yes ☐ No

Menstruating: ☐ Yes ☐ No

Ovulating: ☐ Yes ☐ No

Pregnant: ☐ Yes ☐ No

On Antibiotics: ☐ Yes ☐ No

Had Protected Sex: ☐ Yes ☐ No

Had Unprotected Sex: ☐ Yes ☐ No

Symptoms

☐ Spotting	☐ Light Bleeding	☐ Moderate Bleeding
☐ Heavy Bleeding	☐ Acne/Breakout	☐ Cramps
☐ Tender/Swollen Breasts	☐ Backache	☐ Headache
☐ Joint Pain	☐ Mood Swings	☐ Anxiety/Depression
☐ Bloating	☐ Constipation	☐ Diarrhea
☐ Fatigue	☐ Dizziness	☐ Nausea/Vomiting
☐ Appetite Changes	☐ Pelvic Pressure	☐ Clots/Bloody Discharge
☐ Sticky Discharge	☐ Creamy Discharge	☐ Egg-White Discharge

☐ Other: _____

Notes

Period Tracker

Cycle Day

1 2 3 4 5 6 7 8 9 10 11 12 13 14 15 16 17 18 19 20 21 22 23 24 25 26 27 28 29 30 31 32 33 34 35 36 37 38 39 40 41 42 43 44 45

Date: _____

Avg. Cycle Length: _____

Basal Body Temp: _____

Birth Control Method: _____

Took Birth Control: ☐ Yes ☐ No

Menstruating: ☐ Yes ☐ No

Ovulating: ☐ Yes ☐ No

Pregnant: ☐ Yes ☐ No

On Antibiotics: ☐ Yes ☐ No

Had Protected Sex: ☐ Yes ☐ No

Had Unprotected Sex: ☐ Yes ☐ No

Symptoms

☐ Spotting   ☐ Light Bleeding   ☐ Moderate Bleeding

☐ Heavy Bleeding   ☐ Acne/Breakout   ☐ Cramps

☐ Tender/Swollen Breasts ☐ Backache   ☐ Headache

☐ Joint Pain   ☐ Mood Swings   ☐ Anxiety/Depression

☐ Bloating   ☐ Constipation   ☐ Diarrhea

☐ Fatigue   ☐ Dizziness   ☐ Nausea/Vomiting

☐ Appetite Changes   ☐ Pelvic Pressure   ☐ Clots/Bloody Discharge

☐ Sticky Discharge   ☐ Creamy Discharge   ☐ Egg-White Discharge

☐ Other: _____

Notes

Period Tracker

Cycle Day

(circular chart with numbers 1 through 45)

Date: _____

Avg. Cycle Length: _____

Basal Body Temp: _____

Birth Control Method: _____

Took Birth Control: ☐ Yes ☐ No

Menstruating: ☐ Yes ☐ No

Ovulating: ☐ Yes ☐ No

Pregnant: ☐ Yes ☐ No

On Antibiotics: ☐ Yes ☐ No

Had Protected Sex: ☐ Yes ☐ No

Had Unprotected Sex: ☐ Yes ☐ No

Symptoms

☐ Spotting	☐ Light Bleeding	☐ Moderate Bleeding
☐ Heavy Bleeding	☐ Acne/Breakout	☐ Cramps
☐ Tender/Swollen Breasts	☐ Backache	☐ Headache
☐ Joint Pain	☐ Mood Swings	☐ Anxiety/Depression
☐ Bloating	☐ Constipation	☐ Diarrhea
☐ Fatigue	☐ Dizziness	☐ Nausea/Vomiting
☐ Appetite Changes	☐ Pelvic Pressure	☐ Clots/Bloody Discharge
☐ Sticky Discharge	☐ Creamy Discharge	☐ Egg-White Discharge

☐ Other: _____

Notes

Period Tracker

Cycle Day

(1)(2)(3)(4)(5)(6)(7)(8)(9)(10)(11)(12)(13)(14)(15)(16)(17)(18)(19)(20)(21)(22)(23)(24)(25)(26)(27)(28)(29)(30)(31)(32)(33)(34)(35)(36)(37)(38)(39)(40)(41)(42)(43)(44)(45)

Date: _____

Avg. Cycle Length: _____

Basal Body Temp: _____

Birth Control Method: _____

Took Birth Control: ☐ Yes ☐ No

Menstruating: ☐ Yes ☐ No

Ovulating: ☐ Yes ☐ No

Pregnant: ☐ Yes ☐ No

On Antibiotics: ☐ Yes ☐ No

Had Protected Sex: ☐ Yes ☐ No

Had Unprotected Sex: ☐ Yes ☐ No

Symptoms

☐ Spotting   ☐ Light Bleeding   ☐ Moderate Bleeding

☐ Heavy Bleeding   ☐ Acne/Breakout   ☐ Cramps

☐ Tender/Swollen Breasts ☐ Backache   ☐ Headache

☐ Joint Pain   ☐ Mood Swings   ☐ Anxiety/Depression

☐ Bloating   ☐ Constipation   ☐ Diarrhea

☐ Fatigue   ☐ Dizziness   ☐ Nausea/Vomiting

☐ Appetite Changes   ☐ Pelvic Pressure   ☐ Clots/Bloody Discharge

☐ Sticky Discharge   ☐ Creamy Discharge   ☐ Egg-White Discharge

☐ Other: _____

Notes

Period Tracker

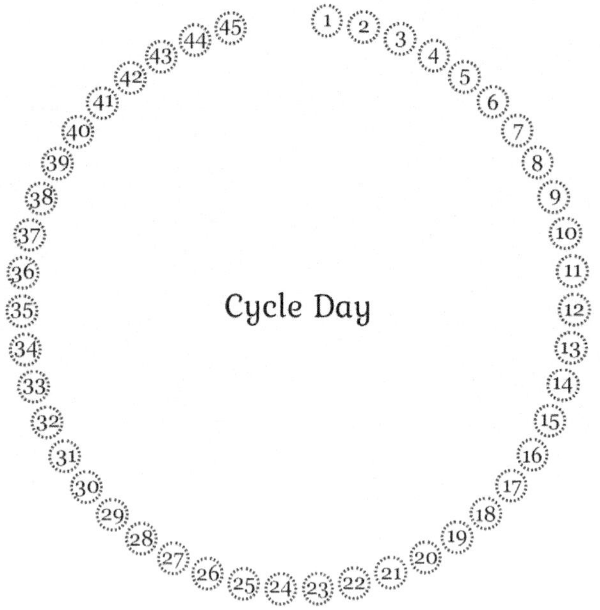

Date: ______________________

Avg. Cycle Length: ______________________

Basal Body Temp: ______________________

Birth Control Method: ______________________

Took Birth Control: ☐ Yes ☐ No

Menstruating: ☐ Yes ☐ No

Ovulating: ☐ Yes ☐ No

Pregnant: ☐ Yes ☐ No

On Antibiotics: ☐ Yes ☐ No

Had Protected Sex: ☐ Yes ☐ No

Had Unprotected Sex: ☐ Yes ☐ No

Symptoms

- ☐ Spotting
- ☐ Light Bleeding
- ☐ Moderate Bleeding
- ☐ Heavy Bleeding
- ☐ Acne/Breakout
- ☐ Cramps
- ☐ Tender/Swollen Breasts
- ☐ Backache
- ☐ Headache
- ☐ Joint Pain
- ☐ Mood Swings
- ☐ Anxiety/Depression
- ☐ Bloating
- ☐ Constipation
- ☐ Diarrhea
- ☐ Fatigue
- ☐ Dizziness
- ☐ Nausea/Vomiting
- ☐ Appetite Changes
- ☐ Pelvic Pressure
- ☐ Clots/Bloody Discharge
- ☐ Sticky Discharge
- ☐ Creamy Discharge
- ☐ Egg-White Discharge
- ☐ Other: ______________________

Notes

Period Tracker

Cycle Day

1 2 3 4 5 6 7 8 9 10 11 12 13 14 15 16 17 18 19 20 21 22 23 24 25 26 27 28 29 30 31 32 33 34 35 36 37 38 39 40 41 42 43 44 45

Date: _____

Avg. Cycle Length: _____

Basal Body Temp: _____

Birth Control Method: _____

Took Birth Control: ☐ Yes   ☐ No

Menstruating: ☐ Yes   ☐ No

Ovulating: ☐ Yes   ☐ No

Pregnant: ☐ Yes   ☐ No

On Antibiotics: ☐ Yes   ☐ No

Had Protected Sex: ☐ Yes   ☐ No

Had Unprotected Sex: ☐ Yes   ☐ No

Symptoms

☐ Spotting   ☐ Light Bleeding   ☐ Moderate Bleeding

☐ Heavy Bleeding   ☐ Acne/Breakout   ☐ Cramps

☐ Tender/Swollen Breasts   ☐ Backache   ☐ Headache

☐ Joint Pain   ☐ Mood Swings   ☐ Anxiety/Depression

☐ Bloating   ☐ Constipation   ☐ Diarrhea

☐ Fatigue   ☐ Dizziness   ☐ Nausea/Vomiting

☐ Appetite Changes   ☐ Pelvic Pressure   ☐ Clots/Bloody Discharge

☐ Sticky Discharge   ☐ Creamy Discharge   ☐ Egg-White Discharge

☐ Other: _____

Notes

Period Tracker

Cycle Day

(circular cycle day tracker numbered 1 through 45)

Date: _____

Avg. Cycle Length: _____

Basal Body Temp: _____

Birth Control Method: _____

Took Birth Control: ☐ Yes ☐ No

Menstruating: ☐ Yes ☐ No

Ovulating: ☐ Yes ☐ No

Pregnant: ☐ Yes ☐ No

On Antibiotics: ☐ Yes ☐ No

Had Protected Sex: ☐ Yes ☐ No

Had Unprotected Sex: ☐ Yes ☐ No

Symptoms

☐ Spotting   ☐ Light Bleeding   ☐ Moderate Bleeding

☐ Heavy Bleeding   ☐ Acne/Breakout   ☐ Cramps

☐ Tender/Swollen Breasts ☐ Backache   ☐ Headache

☐ Joint Pain   ☐ Mood Swings   ☐ Anxiety/Depression

☐ Bloating   ☐ Constipation   ☐ Diarrhea

☐ Fatigue   ☐ Dizziness   ☐ Nausea/Vomiting

☐ Appetite Changes   ☐ Pelvic Pressure   ☐ Clots/Bloody Discharge

☐ Sticky Discharge   ☐ Creamy Discharge   ☐ Egg-White Discharge

☐ Other: _____

Notes

Period Tracker

Cycle Day

(circular diagram numbered 1 through 45)

Date: _____

Avg. Cycle Length: _____

Basal Body Temp: _____

Birth Control Method: _____

Took Birth Control: ☐ Yes ☐ No

Menstruating: ☐ Yes ☐ No

Ovulating: ☐ Yes ☐ No

Pregnant: ☐ Yes ☐ No

On Antibiotics: ☐ Yes ☐ No

Had Protected Sex: ☐ Yes ☐ No

Had Unprotected Sex: ☐ Yes ☐ No

Symptoms

☐ Spotting	☐ Light Bleeding	☐ Moderate Bleeding
☐ Heavy Bleeding	☐ Acne/Breakout	☐ Cramps
☐ Tender/Swollen Breasts	☐ Backache	☐ Headache
☐ Joint Pain	☐ Mood Swings	☐ Anxiety/Depression
☐ Bloating	☐ Constipation	☐ Diarrhea
☐ Fatigue	☐ Dizziness	☐ Nausea/Vomiting
☐ Appetite Changes	☐ Pelvic Pressure	☐ Clots/Bloody Discharge
☐ Sticky Discharge	☐ Creamy Discharge	☐ Egg-White Discharge

☐ Other: _____

Notes

Period Tracker

Cycle Day

(circular chart with days 1–45)

Date: _____

Avg. Cycle Length: _____

Basal Body Temp: _____

Birth Control Method: _____

Took Birth Control: ☐ Yes   ☐ No

Menstruating: ☐ Yes   ☐ No

Ovulating: ☐ Yes   ☐ No

Pregnant: ☐ Yes   ☐ No

On Antibiotics: ☐ Yes   ☐ No

Had Protected Sex: ☐ Yes   ☐ No

Had Unprotected Sex: ☐ Yes   ☐ No

Symptoms

☐ Spotting

☐ Heavy Bleeding

☐ Tender/Swollen Breasts

☐ Joint Pain

☐ Bloating

☐ Fatigue

☐ Appetite Changes

☐ Sticky Discharge

☐ Other:

☐ Light Bleeding

☐ Acne/Breakout

☐ Backache

☐ Mood Swings

☐ Constipation

☐ Dizziness

☐ Pelvic Pressure

☐ Creamy Discharge

☐ Moderate Bleeding

☐ Cramps

☐ Headache

☐ Anxiety/Depression

☐ Diarrhea

☐ Nausea/Vomiting

☐ Clots/Bloody Discharge

☐ Egg-White Discharge

Notes

Period Tracker

Cycle Day

1 2 3 4 5 6 7 8 9 10 11 12 13 14 15 16 17 18 19 20 21 22 23 24 25 26 27 28 29 30 31 32 33 34 35 36 37 38 39 40 41 42 43 44 45

Date: _____

Avg. Cycle Length: _____

Basal Body Temp: _____

Birth Control Method: _____

Took Birth Control:	☐ Yes ☐ No
Menstruating:	☐ Yes ☐ No
Ovulating:	☐ Yes ☐ No
Pregnant:	☐ Yes ☐ No
On Antibiotics:	☐ Yes ☐ No
Had Protected Sex:	☐ Yes ☐ No
Had Unprotected Sex:	☐ Yes ☐ No

Symptoms

☐ Spotting   ☐ Light Bleeding   ☐ Moderate Bleeding

☐ Heavy Bleeding   ☐ Acne/Breakout   ☐ Cramps

☐ Tender/Swollen Breasts   ☐ Backache   ☐ Headache

☐ Joint Pain   ☐ Mood Swings   ☐ Anxiety/Depression

☐ Bloating   ☐ Constipation   ☐ Diarrhea

☐ Fatigue   ☐ Dizziness   ☐ Nausea/Vomiting

☐ Appetite Changes ☐ Pelvic Pressure   ☐ Clots/Bloody Discharge

☐ Sticky Discharge ☐ Creamy Discharge   ☐ Egg-White Discharge

☐ Other: _____

Notes

Period Tracker

Cycle Day

(Circular chart with numbers 1 through 45)

Date: _____

Avg. Cycle Length: _____

Basal Body Temp: _____

Birth Control Method: _____

Took Birth Control:	☐ Yes	☐ No
Menstruating:	☐ Yes	☐ No
Ovulating:	☐ Yes	☐ No
Pregnant:	☐ Yes	☐ No
On Antibiotics:	☐ Yes	☐ No
Had Protected Sex:	☐ Yes	☐ No
Had Unprotected Sex:	☐ Yes	☐ No

Symptoms

☐ Spotting	☐ Light Bleeding	☐ Moderate Bleeding
☐ Heavy Bleeding	☐ Acne/Breakout	☐ Cramps
☐ Tender/Swollen Breasts	☐ Backache	☐ Headache
☐ Joint Pain	☐ Mood Swings	☐ Anxiety/Depression
☐ Bloating	☐ Constipation	☐ Diarrhea
☐ Fatigue	☐ Dizziness	☐ Nausea/Vomiting
☐ Appetite Changes	☐ Pelvic Pressure	☐ Clots/Bloody Discharge
☐ Sticky Discharge	☐ Creamy Discharge	☐ Egg-White Discharge

☐ Other: _____

Notes

Additional Work
ASSIGNMENT PLANNER

○ MONDAY

GOALS THIS WEEK

○ TUESDAY

○ WEDNESDAY

WHAT TO STUDY

○ THURSDAY

○ FRIDAY

EXTRA CREDIT WEEKEND WORK
○ SATURDAY / SUNDAY

Additional Work
ASSIGNMENT PLANNER

○ MONDAY

GOALS THIS WEEK

○ TUESDAY

○ WEDNESDAY

WHAT TO STUDY

○ THURSDAY

○ FRIDAY

EXTRA CREDIT WEEKEND WORK
○ SATURDAY / SUNDAY

Additional Work
ASSIGNMENT PLANNER

○ MONDAY

GOALS THIS WEEK

○ TUESDAY

○ WEDNESDAY

WHAT TO STUDY

○ THURSDAY

○ FRIDAY

EXTRA CREDIT WEEKEND WORK
○ SATURDAY / SUNDAY

A= Above Standards S=	93-97 A	80-82 B	68-69 D+
Meets Standards N=	90-92 A	78-79 C+	62-67 D
Needs Improvement	88-89 B+	73-77 C	60-62 D
98-100 A+	83-87 B	70-72 C	59 & Below F

Track overall daily grade(s)

Week	Monday	Tuesday	Wednesday	Thursday	Friday
1					
2					
3					
4					
5					
6					
7					
8					
9					
10					
11					
12					
13					
14					
15					
16					
17					
18					

Notes

End of the Year Evaluation

Name: _____

Grade/Level: _____ Date: _____

Subjects Studied: _____

_____

_____

Goals Accomplished: _____

_____

_____

_____

Most Improved Areas:_____

_____

_____

_____

Areas of Improvement:_____

_____

_____

Main Curriculum Evaluation	Satisfied			Final Grades
			A= Above Standards	
			S= Meets Standards	
			N= Needs Improvement	
_____	Yes	No	98-100 A+	_____
			93-97 A	
_____	Yes	No	90-92 A	_____
			88-89 B+	
_____	Yes	No	83-87 B	_____
			80-82 B	
_____	Yes	No	78-79 C+	_____
			73-77 C	
			70-72 C	
_____	Yes	No	68-69 D+	_____
			62-67 D	
_____	Yes	No	60-62 D	_____
			59 & Below F	

Most Enjoyed:_____

_____

Least Enjoyed:_____

_____

Made in the USA
Las Vegas, NV
07 December 2023

82255318R00046